# Immunology in the Twentieth Century

# Immunology in the Twentieth Century

# From Basic Science to Clinical Application

Domenico Ribatti
Department of Basic Medical Sciences,
Neurosciences and Sensory Organs,
University of Bari Medical School, Bari, Italy

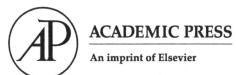

ACADEMIC PRESS

An imprint of Elsevier

Academic Press is an imprint of Elsevier
125 London Wall, London EC2Y 5AS, United Kingdom
525 B Street, Suite 1800, San Diego, CA 92101-4495, United States
50 Hampshire Street, 5th Floor, Cambridge, MA 02139, United States
The Boulevard, Langford Lane, Kidlington, Oxford OX5 1GB, United Kingdom

**Notices**
Knowledge and best practice in this field are constantly changing. As new research and experience broaden our
understanding, changes in research methods, professional practices, or medical treatment may become
necessary.

Practitioners and researchers must always rely on their own experience and knowledge in evaluating and using
any information, methods, compounds, or experiments described herein. In using such information or methods
they should be mindful of their own safety and the safety of others, including parties for whom they have a
professional responsibility.

To the fullest extent of the law, neither the Publisher nor the authors, contributors, or editors, assume any
liability for any injury and/or damage to persons or property as a matter of products liability, negligence or
otherwise, or from any use or operation of any methods, products, instructions, or ideas contained in the
material herein.

**British Library Cataloguing-in-Publication Data**
A catalogue record for this book is available from the British Library

**Library of Congress Cataloging-in-Publication Data**
A catalog record for this book is available from the Library of Congress

ISBN: 978-0-12-816145-6

For Information on all Academic Press publications
visit our website at https://www.elsevier.com/books-and-journals

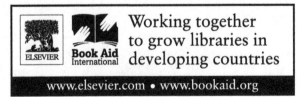

Working together
to grow libraries in
developing countries

www.elsevier.com • www.bookaid.org

*Publisher:* John Fedor
*Acquisition Editor:* Glyn Jones
*Editorial Project Manager:* Pat Gonzalez
*Production Project Manager:* Punithavathy Govindaradjane

Typeset by MPS Limited, Chennai, India

# CONTENTS

# PREFACE

What could be more important than understanding
The very determinants of individuality?

*R.A. Good (1976)*

Each animal species is subjected to continuous selective pressure exerted by the environment and is forced to a slow and constant evolutionary process. Vertebrates provide an ideal environment for development of the most diverse pathogens against whom acts a defensive system represented by the immune system. Giuseppe R. Burgio wrote that: "The biological individuality that must be defined through the phylogeny with the progressive refining of immune functions, starting from the first vertebrates, can also be observed such as a prototype, of an ancestral model of that self-conscious and thoughtful being most frequently used refer to the humanists, philosophers and academics of Human psyche. Certainly it is not possible to talk about self-consciousness regarding the biological being that, unlike other individuals, man has in common with other vertebrates. But it would be tempting to see at least one 'embryo,' a preliminary *experimentum naturae* of self-consciousness in a system like the immune system which maintains the identity of the self continually comparing its contents with those of the world" (1983, p. 508). Only after Ilya Metchnikoff discovered macrophages in 1890 did immunology, which was considered as a branch of bacteriology, acquire the character of an independent science. The origins of new immunology are traced back to discoveries of Landsteiner of blood groups at the beginning of the 20th century.

The relatively simple defense strategies used by invertebrates are based on protective barriers, toxic molecules, and phagocytes that ingest and destroy the pathogens. Also vertebrates depend on these innate immune responses but they can organize more sophisticated defenses defined as adaptive immune responses that are highly specific towards pathogens and provide long-lasting protection.

In the 1940s it was observed that the immunological phenomena are related to the self- and nonself-cells recognition. This mechanism of discrimination between self and nonself allows to the maintenance of the uniqueness of the individual and this is the main function of the immune system. The immune reactions constitute adaptive responses operated by the individual in order to eliminate foreign elements represented by bacteria, virus, parasites, but also tumor cells (immune surveillance). Long before the studies about the involvement of the major histocompatibility complex in the immune response, Sir Thomas Lewis (1881–1945), a British cardiologist, suggested that the rejection mechanism in allo-transplantations, constituted a tool by which the cells of the body can be kept under immune surveillance in order to identify and then eliminate the altered cells with oncogenic potential.

In the clinical settings, the immunology opened new chapters of internal medicine such as autoimmune and immunodeficiency diseases. During autoimmune diseases the immune response is carried out against the self-cells of the organism. In a different way, during immunodeficiency diseases there is a partial or complete defect of immune response that is incompatible with the life.

Immunology contributed to provide a precise connotation and definition about the biological individuality due to the ability acquired by the immune system during the ontogenetic and phylogenetic development to recognize what belongs to ourselves from all that is not. The biological self is substantially the immunological self. Lorenzo Bonomo, one of the founding fathers of clinical immunology in Italy in 1979 wrote that: "A 'mystic' immunology was delineated and 'Immune theology' were discussed about immunological factors such as the complement, the kinin system, both equipped with semimagic properties. It was played on the significance of God (Generator of Diversity) to indicate the randomized natural selection mechanism of the many antibodies of which are endowed with the most evolved organisms such as man" (Bonomo, Schena, 1979, p. 11).

Gilberto Corbellini in the Preface to Tauber (1999, p. IX), wrote that:"Immunology is probably the biomedical science that has gone towards the most extensive cognitive developments in the last four decades, both in terms of the amount of empirical data gained through laboratory research and the conceptual value and the practical implications of these data. From the point of view of fundamental research, the main characterized immunological scientific evolution aspects regarded the definition and the description of adaptive immunity properties and potential of experimental investigation strategies deployed to arrive at the description of physiological processes from which these properties are dependent on [...]. More recently the development of sophisticated systems for physical and biochemical investigation of cells and humoral immunity factors and application of biogenetic technologies led to discoveries whose cognitive significance would be increasingly general biological interest."

For the complexity of cellular interactions and the high specialization of its functions, the immune system is comparable to the nervous system. Niels K. Jerne, a Danish immunologist, Nobel Prize for Medicine in 1984 with Cesar Milstein and Georges Köhler, in 1974 wrote: "These two systems show dichotomies and dualisms. The cells of both systems can receive as well as transmit signals. In both systems, the signals can be either excitatory or inhibitory. The two systems penetrate most other tissues of our body but seem to be kept separate from each other by the so called blood−brain barrier. The nervous system is a network of neurons in which the axon and the dendrites of neuron form synaptic connections with sets of other nervous cells. Lymphocytes are a hundred times more numerous than nervous cells. They do not need connection fibers in order to form a network. As the lymphocytes can move freely, they can interact either by direct encounters or through the antibody molecules they release. The network resides in the ability of these elements to recognize as well as to be recognized. Like for the nervous system, the modulation of the network by foreign signals represents its adaptation to the outside world. Both systems thereby learn from experience and build up a memory that is sustained by reinforcement and that is deposited in persistent network modifications, which cannot be transmitted to our offspring" (Corbellini, 1990, pp. 259−260).

The discovery of immunological synapses has further approached the structural and functional organization of the immune system to that of the nervous system. With the use of high resolution microscope it has been possible to demonstrate the presence of membrane structures similar to nervous synapses also between the immune system cells. In one of the first experiments demonstrating the existence of immunological synapses, Michael L. Dustin, of the Washington

University School of Medicine in St. Louis, used fluorescent dye-labeled proteins inserted inside an artificial membrane. When a T lymphocyte on the opposite side of the membrane begins to interact with these proteins, they assume a synaptic structure.

The host defense mechanisms can go to a series of disturbances, conditioned by genetic or acquired factors, or from iatrogenic causes or secondary factors to other illnesses. In all these conditions it is generally referred to as an "immunocompromised host."

Aged subjects show increased susceptibility to developing infectious and neoplastic diseases and this phenomenon is at least partly related to the alterations that the immune system suffers during aging (immunosenescence).

The adaptive aspects of immunological response are extremely important. In this context, A.L. Tauber underlined that: "Immunology emerged directly from the evolutionary problems posed by the origin of the species and has incorporated both directly and indirectly the central theses of that theory. It seems unambiguous that the immunity concepts that defined this discipline come from debates on evolutionary biology at the end of the 20th century. In addition, despite its deviation, the particular problems of serology and immunochemistry in the first half of the 20th century, immunology has returned to its original program, both for the specific nature of selection theories that represent a common dogma and for the deeper issues that guide its scientific program [...] Regarding the fundamental biologic drama about host defense as a mechanism determined by the evolution to fight the pathogens, an inflammation general theory based on the observation of the simplest" (1999, pp. XXI–XXIII).

Moreover, Corbellini wrote on the adaptive meaning of the immune function: "The power to respond properly and flexibly to the environmental challenges reproduced at individual level a characteristic of life and linked to the dynamic of the biological evolution" (1990, p. 21).

Immunology has greatly benefited from the explosive development of molecular biology incorporating its primary concepts in almost all of its branches and becoming a research field of high heuristic value in biological and medical sciences.

The aim of this book is to delineate synthetically—without the presumption to carry out an exhaustive analysis for which the reader can refer to specialist treatises—the historical profile of some founding elements that have characterized the research in immunological field at the international level during 20th century. In particular, it will examine the problems related to the immune system, to the genetic origins of the immune system, to more frequent pathologies of the immune system, and, lastly, to the interconnection between tumor development and the immune system functioning.

# ACKNOWLEDGEMENT

I am very grateful to Dr. Roberto Tamma for his excellent translation from the Italian version of this book published by CAROCCI EDITORE, Rome, Italy, in 2017.

# CHAPTER 1

# The Antibodies

## 1.1 THE ANTIBODY PRODUCTION

The antibody production mechanism is a central problem of immunology. Research on this mechanism started at the end of 19th century, when the Louis Pasteur theory, according to which the disease causative agents are germs, was officially accepted. Several groups began to study the reactions between bacterial toxins and "antitoxins" that appear in the serum after the infection. The diphteria bacillus was isolated in 1884 and a few years later it was demonstrated that its culture contained a toxin produced by the same bacillus. The injection into a guinea pig of a fraction of the filtered culture fluid caused his death, while animals injected with nonletal doses of the toxin gradually became resistant to its action.

German bacteriologist Emil A. von Behring (Nobel Prize in 1901 for his discoveries on antidiphterial and antitetanic serums) demonstrated together with his Japanese colleague, Shibasaburo Kitasato, that the serum of vaccinated animals contained serum antitoxin and coined for these substances the term Antikörper, or antibodies. In the following years, Belgian physician Jules Bordet, professor of bacteriology and virology at the University of Brussels (Nobel Prize in 1919) demonstrated that antibodies-mediated bactericidal activity required the presence of a thermo-stimulant factor (complement) also present in normal serum. In 1899, Bordet demonstrated that if rabbit red blood cells were injected into the guinea pig, the serum of this one becomes capable of inducing hemolysis in the rabbit red blood cells; hemolytic capacity was destroyed by heating at 56°C for 30 min and reintegrated by the addition of fresh serum of guinea pig not treated with rabbit red blood cells. In 1889, Paul Ehrlich and the pathologist Julius Morgenroth (1871−1924) confirmed these observations and defined as a complement supplementing the nonspecific factor present in normal serum, which was able to completing the hemolytic action of immune sera.[1]

*Immunology in the Twentieth Century*. DOI: https://doi.org/10.1016/B978-0-12-816145-6.00001-9

In 1890, von Behring and Ehrlich[2] published an article describing a technique for measuring antidiphtheria antibodies in the same preparations used by Behring, allowing standardization and thus making serum safe for clinical practice. Ehrlich's quantitative observations demonstrated that the immune response was equivalent to the proliferation of antibodies following contact with an infectious agent.[3]

In 1893 Hans Büchner, a German biochemist, hypothesized that the organism was able to rework the antigen converting it into the specific antibody. Ehrlich was the first to demonstrate that the biological meaning of immune response went beyond the protection from infections and to obtain from rabbits antibody antimilk and egg albumen proteins. He coined the term *horror autotoxicus* to indicate that vertebrates do not produce antibodies directed against one or more of the individual's own proteins, laying the groundwork to explain the difference between *self* and *not-self*. In 1900, Ehrlich proposed the side chains theory into the Cronian Lecture titled "On immunity, with special reference to cell life" to explain antibodies production. The theory hypothesized that a white blood cell had membrane receptors with side chains able to chemically bind the foreign substances. The bond induced the cells to produce many copies of the bound receptor which as antitoxins (antibodies) were transferred into the blood circulation and neutralized toxins.

The side chains theory was based on the assumption that the specificity of the interaction between antigen and antibody was discrete and absolute, in other words the interaction between the antibody molecular structure and the antigen would depend on a complementary stereo adaptation, precise and exclusive, and the chemical reaction dynamic was governed by strong chemical bonds (covalent) (Corbellini, 1996, pp. 256–7).

Ehrlich theory postulated that the antibodies were produced before antigens exposure. This theory was no longer acceptable when it was possible to demonstrate that antibodies against any lab chemically synthesized substance could be formed although no previous exposure had occurred, and it was assumed that the antibodies would be synthesized using the antigen as a template. Franco Celada (1992, p. 13) highlighted that the Ehrlich theory suggests the natural appearance and without any external informational intervention, of different antibody structures in the same cell and the selection of those able to bind to the antigen. The selected structure would then be reproduced in many copies. His contemporary immunologists did not accept the Ehrlich's suggested idea and for over half a century prevailed the innate preference for an explanation that attributed to the antigen the ability to initiate the lymphocytes to antibody-specificity being produced from themselves and from the daughter cells. This attitude had reduced immunology to the last bastion of Lamarckian inheritance.

In 1906, in Germany, Ernest P. Pick, an experimental Czechoslovakian pathologist, together with Friedrich P. Obermayer, an Austrian physician and chemist, demonstrated that when chemical groups containing iodine and nitrate are attached to a protein, its antigenic properties were deeply modified. The Austrian Karl Landsteiner, when he was working at the Rockefeller Institute for Medical Research, put the antigenic proteins at his disposal into contact with a wide variety of chemical groups derived from both pathogenic microbes or synthesized in test tubes (synthetic dyes or haptens)[4] and demonstrated that every molecule induced the formation of a different antibody, so confirming the observations of Pick and Obermayer.

*Since almost nothing was known about the antibody biochemical features but it was possible to induce the organism to react against any foreign chemical structure as long as it was adequately presented, it was intuitive for the immunochemists that the production of a specific antibody occurred under the direct or indirect guidance of the antigen, i.e., the antigen would play an instructive role, acting as a template for the building of antibody structure of recognition (Corbellini, 1996, p. 258).*

The clear result of this was that an animal was able to synthesize a wide (unlimited) set of antibodies but at the same time it was difficult to think that each white blood cell could produce such a large number of side chains. The antibodies present in the serum of an animal immunized by a specific antigen are polyclonal since they constitute the secretion product of different clones of B-lymphocyte each able to produce immunoglobulins (Ig) with peculiar characteristics as to the iso- and idiotype. Polyclonal antibodies have presented numerous limitations mainly related to the heterogeneity of antibody preparation obtained at different times.

These problems have been overcome by the hybridoma technology by which homogeneous populations of antibodies with a defined specificity can be obtained. These antibodies have been termed monoclonal as they are produced by a single cell clone. The revolutionary procedure for obtaining monoclonal antibodies was described by Georges Köhler and Cesar Milstein,[5] Nobel Prize in Medicine in 1984. These authors demonstrated that the fusion between malignant plasma cell and lymphoid cell generated as a result some cells called hybridoma cells that acquired both the properties of a myeloma cell[6] to undergo infinite replication cycles and the characteristic of the immune lymphoid cell to secrete antibodies.[7]

Köhler and Milstein carried out the fusion between myeloma cells and spleen lymphocytes of a mouse after its immunization with a particular antigen. Individual hybrid cells can be cloned and each clone can produce strong quantities of identical antibodies directed against a single antigenic determinant. Clones can be kept alive for ever and injected into animals to obtain large-scale monoclonal antibodies. Monoclonal antibodies were used for the analyses of somatic mutations and it was possible to demonstrate that mutations are very rare in IgMs, which correspond to primary response, while they are common in antibodies of different classes that correspond to secondary response.

The application of murine monoclonal antibodies in humans leads to at least three principal limitations: (1) they are immunogenic; (2) show a relatively short half-life; and (3) have a poor murine antibodies Fc region recognition by the human effector mechanisms. The development of a series of experimental approaches allowed the transforming of a murine immunoglobulin into a chimeric form (part from human and part from mice), and ultimately totally human, allowing its therapeutic use.

With the so-called humanization, it is possible to selectively replace as much as possible of the murine antibody molecule, including the antigen binding regions, with human proteins. The completely human antibodies production has been possible through the development of *phage-display* platforms and recently by means of genetically modified mice. The validity of this innovative pharmacological approach is confirmed since more than 30 monoclonal antibodies approved by the United States (FDA, Food and Drug Administration) and European (EMA, European Medical Agency) regulatory authorities are present today and about 500 more are being developed. At present the monoclonal antibodies are used in many clinical fields including oncology, hematology, rheumatology, immunology, and most recently the cardiovascular field.

## 1.2 THE ANTIBODIES STRUCTURE

In 1926, Lloyd D. Felton (1885–1953) an American immunologist together with his colleague George H. Bailey determined the protein structure of antibodies, which was confirmed through quantitative and qualitative studies of antigen–antibody complex precipitation reactions carried out by Michael Heidelberg and Forrest E. Kendall.

In 1938, Arne Tiselius, a Swedish Biochemist and Nobel Prize in Chemistry in 1948, and US Elvin Kabat, one of the founding fathers of quantitative immunocytochemistry, demonstrated that the serum electrophoresis allowed the separation of the globulins into three bands ($\alpha$, $\beta$, $\gamma$), and they established that antibodies were contained in the $\gamma$ fraction, the one that migrated more slowly. Following this observation, the term gammaglobulins was used as an antibody synonym. Subsequently, since it resulted that the antibody activity was contained also in $\alpha$ and $\beta$ fractions the World Health Organization (WHO) proposed the term of Ig for all the proteins provided with specific antibody activity. It was also possible to establish that immune serum contained different types of antibodies which were subdivided into five classes, Ig G, M, A, D, E on the basis of the different functional and structural characteristics. The basic distinction is based on the existence of class antigens, located in heavy chains (H). These classes depend on different portions of the heavy chain polypeptide, portions that possess antigenic activity by constituting an antibody molecule own epitopes.[8] Some Ig also have additional polypeptides and some of them form five unit oligomeric associations each consisted of heavy and light coupled chains.

In 1956, at the Pasteur Institute in Paris, the French biologist Jacques Oudin (1916–83) discovered the allotypic markers that are the individual specificity of antibody populations within the species, and the Swedish immunogenicist Rune Grubb (1920–98) described the human allotypes. It was possible to demonstrate that the intraspecific antigenic determinants located into the antibodies were genetically determined, i.e., the antigenic differences reflected the primary structural differences of antibodies.

In 1959, the British biochemist Rodney Porter (1917–85), together with the US biologist Gerald E. Edelman (1929–2014), Nobel prize in Medicine in 1972, whilst treating the rabbit antibodies with papaine, broke a monomeric immunoglobulin into three fragments, two of them with the same molecular weight of about 50.000 Da, defined as fragment antigen binding (fab), each containing a site for the combination with the antigen, and the other as crystallizable fragment (fc), with an analogue molecular weight, responsible for numerous effective functions such as complement activation, distribution of Ig in the various compartments of the body, cross-linking of the placental barrier, and catabolism of the whole molecule. The resolution of Ig structure was obtained by establishing the relationship between the polypeptide chains identified by Edelman and the papaine digestion products obtained by Porter.

In 1959, Edelman demonstrated that the reduction with mercaptoethanol in the presence of urea induced the break of 15 disulfide bounds in a monomeric Ig molecule with the separation of four polypeptide chains, two described as heavy, each made of 440 amino acids, and two as light (L) chains, each made of 220 amino acids, with different molecular weights of 55.000 and 23.000 Da, respectively. In 1962, the English biochemist J.B. Fleischman, utilizing mercaptoethanol as a reduction reagent in association with acetamide iodine as agent alchilant, obtained the subdivision of Ig into four polypeptide soluble chains, separable into two fractions by Sephadex-G75 gel-filtation.

In 1963, the US immunologist Henry Kunkel (1916−83) recognized the existence of an Ig marker located in the recognition regions that indicated the antigen specificity of the single antibody, and in 1966 Oudin and M. Michel defined this serological feature as "Idiotypic specificity."

In 1965, Norbert Hilschmann and Lyman C. Craig of Rockfeller University and Frank W. Putman of the University of Florida for the first time sequenced the light chains of a Bence Jones[9] myeloma protein, demonstrating that it consisted of 214 amino acids, and that the polypeptide chains of an antibody were constituted by constant regions (C) and variable regions (V) corresponding to the antigen combination site. It resulted that the Bence Jones proteins obtained from several multiple myeloma patients presented different amino acid sequences and the differences were with regard to the first half of polypeptide chain. In this way it was possible to divide the light chain into a variable region (amino acids 1–108) and into a constant region (amino acids 109–214).

In 1969, Gerald E. Edelman described for the first time the IgG structure derived from a myeloma patient and introduced the concept of the domain. The Ig molecule was composed of 110 amino acid residues. In 1974, Edelman wrote: "In the last decade, the immunology has been extremely modified by two fundamental transformations: the clonal selection theory and the chemical analysis of antibodies structure" (Corbellini, 1990, p. 225).

In the early 1970s, T.T. Wu and Elvin A. Kabat of Columbia University studied the amino acid sequences of the human and animal light chain variable regions and demonstrated that they contained three hypervariable regions in which sequences varied more than the rest of the variable region. The hypervariable sequences included 25 of the 110 amino acid units of the light chain variable region and 30 of the 120 amino acid units of the heavy chain variable region.

Subsequently, the advances in immunochemistry have made it possible to clarify how an antibody molecule adapts to an antigen and has provided much information on the evolution of antibody structure.

## 1.3 THE MOLECULAR BASIS OF ANTIBODIES DIVERSITY

To explain how it was possible produce a repertoire of different antibodies, in 1959, Lenderberg[10] conceived a theory based on the somatic mutation of the antibody polypeptide segments. By contrast, the US immunologist David W. Talmage (1919–2014) believed that all antibody repertoire was already contained in the genome.

In 1965, the US immunologist William J. Dreyer (1928–2004) and his colleague Joe C. Bennett (1935) proposed the hypothesis of two genes codifying a polypeptide chain, according to which a somatic recombination of the antibody chain variable and constant region genes occurred, hypothesizing that more than one gene could be implied in the codification of a polypeptide chain and that the genome would not be kept unaltered during the ontogenesis and the differentiation but was subjected to a reorganization.

During the 1970s it was clarified that the diversity in the antibody repertoire derives from the somatic recombination of a restricted number (about 500) of genes codifying the variable, diversity (D), junction (J), and constant regions of the antibodies. Genes codifying these protein segments are able to combine with each other in a relatively casual mode during the B lymphocyte differentiation, giving rise to antibody molecules with about $10^{10}-10^{12}$ several recombination sites.

In 1976, Susumu Tonegawa (1939), a Japanese biologist and Nobel Prize winner in 1987, and his colleague Nobumichi Hozumi (1945), working at Basel Institute of Immunology applying the recombinant DNA techniques, demonstrated the random combination of the gene segments codifying the antibody molecules. They showed that the genes codifying the light chain constant and variable regions are fragmented and the genetic information is distributed in distinct segments relatively distant with each other of the same chromosome. They discovered the "somatic recombination" of genes during the differentiation, and demonstrated that the arrangement of the light chain genes is different in embryonic and antibody producing cells, which means that genes are scrambled during the development. Through the recombination and mutation mechanisms it is possible to generate a potential diversity of about 18 billion antibodies.

In 1979, Tonegawa and the US geneticist Philip Leder (1934) described the principal mechanism generating the antibody diversity at light chain levels through the recombination of a genic segment termed as variable and a portion of the junction. The genic sequences coding the variable and constant regions are grouped through a tiny gene segment, termed J (junction), which codifies about 10 amino acids belonging to the terminal variable region end (coded for the V-J set). Once they are rearranged, these segments constitute the gene of the structure coding the light chain.

In 1982, Tonegawa demonstrated that even a heavy chain was present at another genic segment (dh) which participated to the formation of the variable portions. During the heavy chains synthesis the rearrangements does not occur with two but with three types of genic segments (V, D, and J) and the additional segments D (diversity) alternate with V and J. Somatic recombination would be the basis of the diversity of antibodies before assembly with the antigen, whereas the point mutations regarded the immune memory cells.

## 1.4 HOW AN ANTIGEN INFLUENCES THE ANTIBODY STRUCTURE

The main theories about the antibody-poiesis have been classified by Lederberg into two categories:

1. Instructive (of direct and indirect mold);
2. Selective.

As regards the first, the antigen induces the competent cells to synthesize antibodies through a combinatory site complementary to their own structure. As regards the second, the antigen selects and selectively stimulates cells already provided with specific synthetic capacity.

*Direct template theory.* In 1930 Friedrich Breinl and Felix Haurowitz of the University of Prague and in 1932 Stuart Mudd and Jerome Alexander of the University of Pennsylvania argued that the antibodies were synthesized following direct contact with the corresponding antigens, taking chemical shape and affinity complementary to the antigen ("The antibody molecule grows only if it meets the spatial and chemical requirements of the antigen-protoplasm interface, where the synthesis is performed," Mudd, 1932, p. 423)[11] In this way, antibody specificity was explained and that antibodies against any type of substance can be produced, including the synthetic ones.

In 1940, the US chemist (1901−94), Linus Pauling, believed that all the antibodies had the same amino acid composition and sequence and that they were directly synthesized starting from a template represented from the antigen. Moreover, he believed that a wide range of bond specificity could derive from the antibody molecule folding in different ways, making it a particular steric disposition modeled on the antigenic and complementary sites: "All the antibody molecules differ from the normal globulin only in chains configuration, i.e., the way which the chains fold into the chains" (Pauling, 1940, p. 2643). The antibody specificity would therefore be the consequence of the molecular shape and not of the primary structure. In 1954, Pauling obtained the Nobel Prize for Chemistry for his research about the nature of the chemical bond and for his application in explanation of the complex substances structure. With his controversial and philanthropic spirit, he fought for the ban on atomic experiments and in 1962 he had a second Nobel Prize, this time for peace.

Gordon L. Ada, an Australian biochemist (1922–2012), and Gustav Nossal, an Australian biologist (1931) wrote in 1987: "These discussions on the antibodies formation mechanisms happened before the advent of molecular biology in fifties; they were based more on the theory than on experimental data" (in Celada, 1992, p. 31). The theory of the direct template was rejected in 1964 when E. Haber demonstrated that the denatured antibodies when renatured in a physiologic medium, recovered the original antigen specificity.

*Indirect template theory.* Regarding this theory—formulated in 1941 by Frank MacFarlane Burnet,[11] an Australian researcher who worked at Walter and Elizabeth Hall Institute for Medical Research of Melbourne, in his book *The Production of Antibodies*, republished in 1949 with the virologist Frank J. Fenner—the antigen would only durably change the structure of the protein-formation system, through an intermediate that could survive long after the disappearance of the antigen and that was inheritable from daughter cells. The indirect template could be represented from enzyme induced by the antigen. For Burnet and Fenner, who conceived the immune response in Darwinian terms,[12] believing that the antibody producing cells were subjected to a mutation and selection, the antigens had the functions to "instruct" the adaptive enzymes that after the recognizing of antigen configuration, were able to synthesize the antibody also without the presence of the antigen. When an antigen goes throughout an antibody-poietic cell it undergoes adaptive enzymatic modifications so that the synthesized antibody is built as an antigen model. The adaptive enzymatic modifications would be stable for cells and would be transmitted to the progeny.

*Clonal selection theory.* In 1955, the Danish Niels Kaj Jerne published an article entitled The Natural Selection Theory of Antibody Formation, in which he proposed some criticisms to the Burnet and Fenner template theory. The template theory was not able to explain the exponential increase in antibodies production during the first steps of immunological response; the strong increase when the animal contacted the same antigen for the second time; the immunological tolerance phenomenon which prevents an animal producing antibodies against itself and which can be acquired for foreign antigens with which the organism entered in contact before birth, or shortly thereafter. Jerne thought that the antibody already exists before encountering the antigen because the normal serum contains only not-specific antibodies and he cited a paper from Robert Doerr of the University of Basel referring to the natural antibodies produced independently from the antigen stimulation. The canonical immunological response occurs when an antigen binds an antibody and the antigen–antibody complex interacts with lymphocytes inducing the synthesis and release of large amounts of the same specific antibody.

In 1957–59, David W. Talmage, of Colorado University at Denver, claimed that the different mixtures made of a defined number of antibodies with variable specificities were able to differentiate a larger number of different antigens. Ada and Nossal wrote: "Jerne and Talmage in their two publications laid the foundations of the clonal selection theory for antibodies production. Burnet had the task of realizing an organic synthesis of the new concepts developed through his considerations with Fenner" (in Celada, 1992, p. 32).

Between 1957 and 1959 Burnet developed the clonal selection theory showing that the binding of an antigen with an antibody triggers cell multiplication and the clones derived from a cell can produce only one type of the same antibody. The exponential increase in antibody synthesis following antigen stimulation is due to the exponential increase in the number of cells producing those antibodies. Burnet in his article published in 1957, in which he proposed a variant of Jerne's model, wrote:

"In this sense the differential proliferation will be started from those clones among all that will present reactive sites that correspond to the determinants present on the antigen used. Descendants will include plasmocyte-like forms and lymphocytes that react to the same functions of parental forms. The practical result will be a change in the globulin molecules composition in order to provide an excess of molecules able to react with the antigen."

Immune tolerance was explained as a deletion of an entire cell clone that may occur before or after birth. Burnet formulated the hypothesis that during prenatal development all antigens are autoantigen. Recognition of an epitope during gestation would lead to a mechanism of clonal suicide that would lead to the elimination of all potentially self-reactive clones. This would be the main mechanism of inducing tolerance to self-antigens that would make lymphoid cells able to distinguish self from not-self. Autoimmune diseases would appear as a consequence of exposure after births to autoantigens that were still segregated during gestation.

Burnet and Fenner developed the theory that the potential antigens, which react with the lymphocytes during their development in the immature immunological stage, can suppress any future response again to that antigen when the animal will be immunologically mature.

In 1959 in Melbourne, Gustav Nossal, then a young scholar of that university, and Joshua Lederberg of the University of Wisconsin, who spent a few months in the Burnet Laboratory with a Fullbright grant, immunized rats by two different flagellar antigens and demonstrated that while the number of cells producing antibodies against one type of flagellum were increased, no cells were able to produce antibodies against both types (one cell, one antibody). This is the direct testimony of Nossal:

> By the use of very thin needles we tried to break the tissue to obtain a single cells suspension; we then introduced these cells, one by one, in droplets of a volume not greater than one millionth of milliliters. We surrounded the droplets with a thin layer of mineral oil to avoid the evaporation and after a short incubation we added five to ten bacteria with the same flagella and in rapid movement to each droplet. If the bacteria appeared immobilized when observed by microscope indicating the presence of a type of antibody, bacteria with the other type of flagellum were inserted. (in Celada, 1992, p. 34)

By means of this experiment, Burnet was able to convince more researchers of the validity of the clonal selection theory.

This experiment clearly demonstrated that a cell produces a specific antibody type but does not indicate through which mechanism. The variety of antibodies produced by the immune system is estimated at about 10–100 billion, far above the number of our genes, about 25,000. The problem would be faced and resolved by Japanese Susumu Tonegawa, who for his discoveries won the Nobel Prize in 1987.

In 1963, Henry G. Kunkel and colleagues at the Rockefeller Institute for Medical Research, and Jacques Oudin of the Pasteur Institute of Paris, obtained the antibodies production after exhibiting laboratory animals to antigens. The initial antibody (Ac1) isolated from the animal serum and then injected into another animal induced the synthesis of a second antibody (Ac-2) that specifically binds only to the Ac-1 antibody, recognizing the individuality. Oudin coined the term "Ac-1 idiotype" to define the unique antigenic determinants present on this antibody and "antiidiotype antibody" for Ac-2 antibody produced in response to the idiotype.

The concepts of idiotype and antiidiotype were resumed and developed by Niels Jerne who gave them a strong heuristic value. Jerne elaborated the theory of the "idiotypic network" that integrates the theory of clonal selection because an antigenic stimulation induces the clonal expansion of B lymphocytes that produce antibodies equipped of antigenic determinants (idiotypes). The organism then develops some antiidiotype antibodies, and Jerne's immune response would be regulated through a series of interactions between the idiotype and the antiidiotype, since the expression of each idiotype would be controlled by the correspondent antiidiotype that is able to selectively inhibit the idiotype production. Jerne suggested that, since idiotype–antiidiotype interactions are repeated infinitely, an alteration could propagate through the idiotypes network. More recently, it has been demonstrated that the interactions are limited to a finite number. Numerous experimental models have confirmed in humans the existence of antibodies with antiidiotype specificity involved in regulating the immune response.

As Corbellini emphasized (1990, pp. 49–50):

*By the introduction of 'paratope', 'epitope' and 'idiotype', Jerne means to get rid of the linguistic weight of classic immunology represented mainly by the words 'antibody' and 'antigen'. These conceptually bind the system functionality to its interaction with the outside, while it is logically plausible that the antibodies diversity repertoire can be dynamically maintained through idiotype antiidiotype recognition, i.e., by interaction between the antibodies combination sites, which can function as paratopes (antigen recognizing sites) and epitopes (determinant recognized by antibody sites).[13] At this stage it is hard to tell what is the interior and the exterior, or 'the self' and 'the not self,' but a network of interactions among autologous molecular groups, representing the system activity, its 'internal life'. The concept of 'repertoire' which must also include the idiotypes together with the epitopes, the 'dualism' problem, as the existence of two types of cells and of the double recognizing aspect of the system, and the issue of the 'suppression' validate for Jerne the existence of a formal network of interactions in the immune system.*

The Jerne's theory has allowed a new and more convincing interpretation of etiopathogenesis in autoimmune diseases. In myasthenia gravis, an idiotype can react with the acetylcholine receptor, blocking it and destroying it. In Graves' disease, an autoimmune pathology characterized of an abnormal development of thyroid, an antiidiotype can exercise the opposite effect mimicking the thyroid hormone structure and so binding its cell membrane receptor and stimulating the thyroid. Also in the case of rheumatoid arthritis and systemic lupus erythematosus there are evidences of an antiidiotype involvement. It has been demonstrated that rheumatoid factors in the rheumatoid arthritis and anti-DNA antibodies in lupus express a common idiotype in each patient and the antiidiotype would contribute to triggering the disease, stimulating the production of antibodies in serum patients.

## ENDNOTES

1. While at first the complement was believed a single substance, further researches demonstrated that it is composed of several components. The first observation in this sense was made in 1907 by Adolfo Ferrata, a famous hematologist and responsible for research in all areas of hematology, who noted that if the guinea pig serum is dialyzed, its complementary activity disappears. At the same time a precipitate is formed, and neither the precipitate nor the supernatant are active individually, but the activity reappears by gathering the two fractions after the precipitate solubilzation. The complement consists of at least two fractions, one precipitable by dialysis and the other not.

2. Born in Sterhlen, Silesia on March 14, 1854, Ehrlich after high school enrolled at the Faculty of Medicine first in Wroclaw and then in Strasbourg, Freiburg, and Leipzig. In 1878, he obtained a PhD discussing a thesis on the theory and practice of animal tissues staining. After becoming an assistant at Berlin's Medical Clinic, and then a free professor in 1887, Ehrlich was appointed as associate professor at the University of Berlin. In 1890, he was named as

    Assistant at the new Institute of Infectious Diseases by Robert Koch (1843–1910), bacteriologist and German microbiologist. In 1896, he became the director of the new Institute for the Control of Therapeutic Sera in Berlin.

    It was here that Ehrlich developed a procedure to accurately determine the antitoxin content and for this reason he can be considered as the founding father of standardization of sera. Moving to Frankfurt in 1899, he committed himself to chemotherapy, a term coined by himself and with which he indicated the chemical fight against pathogens.

    In 1908, Ehrlich shared the Nobel Prize with Ilya Metchnikoff, a Russian biologist and immunologist who described for the first time the phagocytosis mechanism. Ehrlich's greatest reputation derives from arsenic-based antisyphilis drugs: the Salvarsan, produced by Hoechst since 1910, and the Neosalvarsan that followed shortly afterwards. For 30 years, until the introduction of penicillin, these drugs remained the main cure for syphilis. Ehrlich died in Bad Hamburg on August 20, 1915. He was buried in the Jewish cemetery of Frankfurt.

3. As Frank M. Burnet (1967, pp. 19–20) highlighted: "Ehrlich was first of all an organic chemist and was particularly impressed by the quantitative regularity that allowed him to titling the toxin and the antitoxin in a reasonably accurate manner. Overall, these were the conclusions on which it was aimed : (1) penetration of toxin into the body caused a stimulus to produce the corresponding antitoxin; (2) that antitoxin was chemically combined with toxin, neutralizing its activity."

4. In 1921, Landsteiner observed that it was possible to obtain modifications in the antigenic specificity of a protein conjugating it with diazotized aromatic amines, in order to introduce well known structures into the molecule.

When the diazotized obtained proteins with known determinants were inoculated in animals of different species, antibodies were produced able to specifically react with the diazotized protein but not with the native protein. Landstainer introduced the haptens concept, that is the production of specific antibodies induced by molecules fixed to a protein and then injected into organism. In experiments with synthesized molecules that probably did not exist in nature, Landsteiner observed immune responses that demonstrated that the organism had an innate ability to recognize specific molecules.

5. Köhler (1946−95) was a german biologist who in the 1970s at the Medical Research Council of Cambridge began the collaboration with Milstein (1927−2002), a British nationalized Argentine biochemist.

6. Multiple myeloma is a cancer of the plasma cells, terminal differentiated elements of B lymphocytes. The serum electrophoresis of a patient with myeloma shows a monoclonal peak and the reduction of the normal gamma-globulins. Myeloma is the best evidence that every plasma cell produces only one type of antibody.

7. The scientific paper that described for the first time the process of monoclonal antibodies production, signed by Köhler and Milstein, was published on "Nature" in August 1975 without the impact that was attributed to it later. In fact, 3 years passed before the scientific community realized its importance. Milstein also saw a refusal to patent the discovery from the British institutions.

8. The portions of the antibody hypervariable regions which contact the antigen are termed paratopes and the antigen portion in contact with the paratope is defined as the epitope or antigenic determinant. Most antigens have various antigenic determinants that can stimulate antibody production, T cell specific responses, or both. There are five classes of antibodies in mammals: IgA, IgD, IgE, IgG, and IgM, each with its own heavy chain class, respectively $\alpha$, $\delta$, $\varepsilon$, $\gamma$, and $\mu$. Even in the absence of antigen stimulation, a human can produce $10^{12}$ different antibody molecules. Both light and heavy antibody molecule chains can be subdivided into constant regions, in which the sequence of amino acids is essentially invariable, and variable regions. The variability of the latter resides mostly in small portions called hypervariable. X-ray crystallography studies performed by Mario L. Amzel at National Institutes of Health have highlighted polypeptide chains that are folded in such a way that the hypervariable regions of each chain interact to form a space or bag in which the binding to the antigen occurs.

9. These proteins found in urine were observed in 1847 by Henry Bence Jones at London Guy's Hospital for the first time, and since then are known as Bence Jones proteins. It is possible to obtain them from myeloma patients urine samples and they constituted the first Ig components whose aminoacidic sequence was analyzed.

10. Joshua Lederberg (1925−2008) was a US microbiologist. After a PhD in microbiology at Yale University in 1948, he started along his career as a researcher that led him in 1958 to achieve the Nobel Prize for Medicine "for discoveries on genetic recombination and the organization of bacteria genetic material."

11. Burnet has been involved in genetic recombination in animal viruses. He discovered that the pathogen Q fever antigen is a rickettsia (*Coxiella burneti*), he performed researches in bacteriophages and he developed for the first time ax experimetal method for virus culture in chick embryos.

12. Darwinian ascendancy of Burnet's thinking was emphasized by Ada and Nossal when they wrote: "Burnet conceived the immune response as a kind of Darwinian microcosm. The antibodies producing cells as a organism into an ecosystem, are subjected to mutation and selection; the most suitable ones survive and the suitability in this case, is literally the adaption between an antibody produced by an organism cell and the antigen" (in Celada, 1992, p. 33).

Yet, according to Edelman: "The clonal selection system is similar to the natural selection that occurs during the evolution of vertebrates in which immunity is manifested. However, it should be highlighted that these processes differ for a number of key features. The most evident is the time scale on which the two types of selection work: days and months one, millions of years the other. Moreover, it is clear that the clonal selection system is simpler: only one type of molecular object and only a few types of cells are implicated in the process, and the selection takes place within the somatic cells of an organism, rather than among organisms" (in Corbellini, 1990, p. 237).

13. Each antibody region contains antigenic determinants which can stimulate the antibodies production. The constant regions have determinants that are identical in antibodies belonging to the same class and constitute the isotype of an antibody. Constant regions also have determinants that are identical in all individual antibodies, but different in antibodies from different individuals, and which constitute the allotype of an antibody. Determinants only present in the variable regions at the combination site are the idiotype.

# CHAPTER 2

# The Cells of Immunity

In 1882—84, Ilya Metchnikoff was the first to consider immunity as an active response of the organism to a pathogen and to infection. In 1882, he executed the famous experiment in which he observed the phagocytes attacked the thorn of a rose that were placed between the transparent starfish larvae. These are his words:

> I was resting from the shock of the events that provoked my resignation from the university and I was dedicating with enthusiasm to research in the splendid scenery of the Strait of Messina. A day [...] I remained alone with my microscope, observing the life in mobile cells of a transparent starfish larvae, when a new thought suddenly crossed the brain. I understood that similar cells could serve in the defense of the organism against intruders. Feeling that there was in this something interesting, I felt so excited that I started to go forward and back to the room and went also on the beach to collect my thought. I told myself that if my assumption was true, a splinter introduced into the body of a starfish larvae, lacking of blood vessels or a nervous system, would be soon surrounded by mobile cells as it is observed in a man who has a thorn in his finger. It was soon done. There was a small garden where we made a Christmas tree a few days before; I took some thorns from it and put them under the skin of some beautiful transparent like water starfish larvae. I was too excited to sleep that night awaiting the result of my experiment and the next morning, very soon, I was assured of its success. That experiment constituted the basis of phagocyte theory, the development of which I dedicated the next 25 years of my life.

Metchnikoff made a distinction between microphages and macrophages as mediators of cell immune response. The microphages include the blood circulating granulocytes, whereas the macrophages include the reticulo-endothelial system cells, which are distinguished as immobile (reticular cells, Kupffer cells, and spleen sinus cells) and mobile (histiocytes and adventitial blood vessel cells). How wrote Tauber (1999, p. 5):

> Metchnikoff was the first in recognizing the true meaning of the phagocyte as inflammatory cell, to define its function in all the main particulars and to formulate a modern concept of the immune process as a particular case of inflammation. He understood that the fight between pathogen and phagocytes was the specific expression of the organism's effort in maintaining its integrity.

Immunology in the Twentieth Century. DOI: https://doi.org/10.1016/B978-0-12-816145-6.00002-0

For Metchnikoff the specific antibodies were produced by micro-phages which stimulated the phagocytosis in phagocytes. He proposed the phagocytosis and cellular immune theory, in contrast to the humoral immunity. In 1988, George H.H. Nuttal, a US bacteriologist (1862–1937) discovered that defibrinated blood had bactericidal activity and asserted that the phagocytic cells removed the bacteria killed by a thermostable substance present in blood. In 1901, Metchnikoff wrote:

> In vertebrates two large categories of white blood cells are found and those belonging to one of them are similar to the invertebrate white blood cells because they also possess a unique big nucleus and an amoeboid protoplasm. They are the blood and lymphatic macrophages, strictly bound to the macro-phages belonging to other organs such as the spleen, lymphatic ganglia and the bone marrow. The other category of vertebrate white blood cells is consti-tuted of small amoeboid cells that are distinguished by their nucleus, which, although unique, is divided into different lobes. They are the microphages, whose main peculiarity, that is the multi-lobed shape of the nucleus, it must be considered as an adaptation to overcome as quickly as possible to the wall of the capillaries or small veins. (The immunity in infectious diseases, in Corbellini, 1990, p. 94)

At the beginning of the 20th century, morphologists observed that some cells took intravenously injected dyes (such as pyrrolo blue, called "vital dyes" because they colored the living cells). The German pathologist Karl A.L. Aschoff (1862–1942) identified in connective tis-sue these cells as macrophages, in the central nervous system as micro-glia, in vascular sinuses as endothelial cells, and in lymphoid organs as reticular cells. Aschoff suggested that these different cell types were implied in host defense through the phagocytosis of foreign agents such as microbes, and collectively grouped them into the so-called endothelial-reticulum system (RES). The term was introduced in 1924 by Aschoff to indicate all cells provided of phagocytic activity. The definition is due to the fact that a main group of cells, the starred spleen and lymph nodes macrophages, formed a reticulum, and that the other cells tapped the dilated sinuses of blood and lymphatic circu-lation. The phagocytes widely distributed in the connective tissue of different organs were defined histiocytes. The vital staining, the incor-poration of staining colloidal micelles and the cytoplasm micelles pre-cipitation were considered as the equivalent of the phagocytic activity performed by these cells. In the RES were included the reticulum cells, the reticuloendothelium of the hemolymphopoietic organs, the sinusoid of liver (Kupffer cells), adrenal and pituitary glands, the free loose connective cells, the splenocytes, and monocytes. Since the vascular endothelium does not have a histiocytic character and the hemolymphopoietic organs lymphoid cells are not endothelial, the name of SRE was replaced by M. Volterra in 1927 with reticulo-histioctyte system (RIS), on the basis of the nonexclusive endothelial origin of such cellular elements. The current definition of mononuclear phagocytes was established at the beginning of the 1960s.

Mononuclear phagocytes represent the example of a cellular population fundamental for natural immunity, which has also gained a central role in acquired immunity. Many functions operated by macrophages are related to the host defense before a specific immunity develops, functions that become much more efficient in sites where an immune response develops.[1] Dendritic cells, skin Langherans cells, liver Kupffer cells, and central nervous system microglia cells share different morphological, biochemical, and functional characteristics with tissue macrophages. The specific functional characteristics of such cells are: the ability to phagocytize microorganisms; the ability to handle antigens and to present them to the lymphocytes; the synthesis of many cytokines and chemokines able to initiate and/or amplify or terminate the inflammatory reaction, to promote the recruitment of inflammatory cells, and to modulate lymphocytic response; and the ability to recognize and destroy neoplastic cells. Numerous experimental evidences indicate that tissue macrophages and other specialized cellular elements derive from circulating monocytes.

These cells are able to modulate the immune response and play a primary role in inducing and maintaining the inflammatory process. They originate in the bone marrow, probably from a common, CD34 positive myeloid precursor, that originates blood monocytes. Subsequently, monocytes migrate to different tissues where they differentiate in specialized cells after the exposure to different microenvironmental factors. Macrophages are virtually present in all organs where they play an important role in immune responses and local inflammation, tissue damage and repair, apoptotic cell clearance, and antineoplastic monitoring.

Numerous experimental studies in animals have shown significant functional differences between the macrophages isolated from different organs. For example, lung alveolar macrophages synthesize larger amounts of cytokines and have a more effective tumoricidal action than the macrophages of the peritoneal cavity. Spleen and thymus isolated macrophages express markers implicated in the antigen presentation and in the T lymphocyte costimulation. These observations suggest that local factors and tissue microenvironment could guide the development and the functional maturation of macrophages towards the predominant activity required in a particular organ.

Tumor-associated macrophages (TAM) are derived from blood monocytes and are recruited by cytokines with chemotactic activity (chemokines) released by tumor cells into the tumor mass. TAM are able to exert cytotoxic activity against tumor cells.

The interactions between mononuclear phagocytes and lymphocytes include the response to signals derived from lymphocytes (chemotactic lymphokines, activation factors) and the interference with lymphocyte functions. The latter may be nonspecific, as the interferon proliferative suppressive effects on lymphocytes,[2] or specific such as the proliferative stimulation and interleukin-1 (IL-1)[3] mediated lymphocyte differentiation and processing and antigen presentation.


## 2.1 LYMPHOCYTES

In a human adult organism there are about $2 \times 10^{12}$ lymphocytes with a mass comparable with a liver or brain. The lymphocytes were described for the first time in England by the British anatomist William Hewson (1739–74), considered as the father of hematology, in a series of works published around 1770 by the Royal Society. In 1879, Paul Ehrlich described the morphology of lymphocytes believing that they were nonmobile elements and apparently lacking of any function.

In 1930, a possible relationship between lymphocytes and immune response was established, highlighting the germinal center in the immunized rats' lymph nodes (Hellman, 1930). In 1935, the antibodies production in the lymph nodes of immunized animals was observed (McMaster and Hudack, 1935). The reevaluation of lymphocyte function as immune organs resulted from the observation that the lymph reflux from an antigen stimulated lymph node contained more antibodies than the afferent one and that the lymphocytes isolated from the same lymph node were capable of producing soluble antibodies in vitro (Ehrlich and Harris, 1942).

The ambiguity about the significance of lymphocytes, which has made them considered from time to time as multipotent stem cells, nutritional cells, or trephocytes, elements able to regulate the development and volume of organs or eliminating autologous aberrant cells, has been maintained. In the 1960s, two significant biological features of lymphocytes were defined, with the demonstration that these cells are responsible for the organism's immunological reactions (Medawar, 1958), and that, following the stimulation with mitogenic substances of plant origin (lectins), lymphocytes are subjected to proliferation and transformation (Nowell, 1960).

The heterogeneity, immune competence and the ability in proliferating and transforming of lymphocytes represented numerous parameters for studying these cells. All the observations are contextualized by a dualistic conception of immunocompetent system, which has been first demonstrated in birds and later extended also to the mammals.

The existence of two types of immune reactions respectively mediated by cells (lymphocytes) and humoral antibodies are related to two different types of lymphocytes, T and B, which are produced and operate in the environment of two different systems, respectively defined thymus-dependent and bursa-dependent (or thymus-independent). The latter depend on "bursa of Fabricius" (cfr. par. 2.3) in the birds whereas in mammals the liver was first recognized as a bursa equivalent organ during the fetal hemopoiesis by Owen in 1974.

In each of the two systems it is considered there is a central compartment (thymus and "bursa of Fabricius," or bursa equivalent organs) as a site of immunocompetent cells maturation and a peripheral compartment represented by T- and B-dependent spleen regions, lymph nodes, lymphoid tissue organized at the level of the wall of digestive and respiratory apparatus to constitute the MALT, or mucosa associated lymphoid tissue, where immunological responses take place.

The application of analysis techniques suitable for functional characteristics of primitive hematopoietic cells has allowed to overcome the classifications based on morphological criteria and to confirm the derivation of all of the blood figurative elements from a multipotent stem cell, the hemangioblast. The stem cells from which the lymphocytes derive were called CFU (colony forming units). The CFU are recognizable with the hemocytoblasts and appear as large cells with numerous well-evident nucleoli and basophilic cytoplasm (Maximov, 1924); they are characterized at the ultrastructural examination by the abundance of polyribosomes distributed throughout the cytoplasm (Edmonds, 1966).

In the course of the ontogeny, the CFU appear initially in the mesenchyme of the yolk sac for migrating into the fetal liver, which constitutes the main hematopoietic organ in the early months of prenatal life. In the following months this role is gradually assumed by the bone marrow that will keep it throughout the postnatal life. In general, it is believed that the stem cell differs in the precursors of the various hematopoietic maturation lines under the influence of microenvironment and humoral stimuli.

The thymus provides the microenvironment for the differentiation of T precursors derived from the bone marrow which interact with the nonlymphoid thymus cells, including the epithelial cortical cells and the medulla thymic lobules cells and other cells able to present the antigen including macrophages and the dendritic cells. Until then it was incorrectly thought that thymus epithelial cells were themselves transformed into lymphocytes, but studies conducted in the 1960s by Malcom AS Moore and John T. Owen at Oxford University, clearly demonstrated that the precursors of T cells originated from the yolk sac.

If an antigen is made highly radioactive, it kills the T cells with which it interacts, while other T cells that recognize other antigens are not damaged. Through this phenomenon that they called "antigenic suicide," the immunologist Australian Anthony Basten (1939) and his collaborators at the Walter and Heliza Institute demonstrated that T cells include different clones.

As a result of the interaction with the epithelial cells, the T cells undergo a polyclonal expansion process. The cells which express at low or intermediate affinity the T receptor versus the major histocompatibility complex molecules (MHC) survive (positive selection).

At a later stage that occurs in the thymus medulla, a part of lymphocytes' potentially autoreactivity is killed by a negative selection mechanism through an apoptotic process. Studies in mouse have shown that when the lymphopoietic activity is higher, the thymus exports only a small amount of its lymphocytic pool. The vast majority of thymocytes (more than 95%) die via apoptosis.

The negative selection determines the elimination of T cell clones which express T receptor at high affinity for MHC autologous molecules and for autoantigens and it is controlled by the AIRE (Autoimmune Regulator) genes, whose alterations could promote the development of autoimmune pathologies. The AIRE gene encodes a transcription factor that controls the expression of tissue-specific antigens by thymic medulla epithelial cells. The ability to express tissue-specific antigens allows the apoptotic elimination of T autoreactive lymphocytes against these antigens, and in the absence of this function, peripheral tissues become targets of autoreactive T lymphocytes clones against specific tissue-specific antigens.

However, since not all autoantigens are presented in the thymus, T autoreactive lymphocytes could circulate in the organism. This has no consequences until autoantigen reaches the spleen or another lymphoid tissue where it activates the T autoreactive lymphocytes which reach a target organ which presents the autoantigen triggering an autodestructive reaction that is the basis of autoimmune pathologies.

At the end of the differentiation process there are two subpopulations of medulla thymocytes expressing CD4 or CD8 surface markers[4] in a mutually exclusive manner and able to enter into the bloodstream. CD4 cells exert helper/inducer functions as they promote the synthesis of immunoglobulins by the B lymphocytes and cooperate in the generation of T cytotoxic cells with restricted MHC lytic capacity. The CD8 cells play a direct cytotoxic activity. About 90% of the CD4 cells and 60%–80% of the CD8 cells are small, with high nucleus cytoplasmic-ratio, and contain one or more Gall bodies, consisting of a combination of lysosomal granules with a lipid droplet.

In mammals, B cells differentiate first in the fetal liver and later in the bone marrow that after birth provides the microenvironment for their differentiation. This process occurs through an adhesive interaction of B cell progenitors with bone marrow reticular cells that synthesize cytokines, such as IL-7, capable of sustaining their growth. B mature lymphocytes following antigen stimulation lose IgD expressed at the membrane level together with IgM and express in sequence other isotypes (IgG, IgA, and IgE). This process is called "isotype switch." During the B cell activation process, memory cells also develop, resulting in faster secondary antibody responses. The last maturation stage of B cells is the plasma B cell that contains large amounts of cytoplasmic antibodies, and their number in the tissues increases in coincidence with the production of antibodies.

The rearrangement of the genes for Ig and the synthesis of Ig is a unique feature of B lymphocytes. Ig and gene rearrangement process is the most important marker for the identification of B lymphocytes and for their differentiation analysis in which we identify at least three stages: pre-B cells, immature B cells, and B mature cells.

In 1965, two works were simultaneously published in "Nature" demonstrating that the proliferating lymphocytes conditioned media contained an unidentified substance able to potentiate the development of lymphocytes in the presence of the antigen (Kasakura and Lowenstein, 1965; Gordon and Mac Lean, 1965). In 1976, Doris A. Morgan, working at the National Cancer Institute in Bethesda, published a paper in "Science" in which he reported that normal T lymphocytes could be cultured without any antigen even for 9 months, provided that conditioned lymphocyte media were added at regular intervals to the cultures (Morgan et al., 1976).

The dualistic concept of the immunocompetent system does not imply a complete dichotomy of the two sectors. The collaboration between the lymphocytes of the two systems and other cell types constitutes the crucial condition for the occurring of many immune responses (Mitechell and Miller, 1968; Miller et al., 1971). The existence of this cooperation was demonstrated by a set of classical experiments performed by Henry N. Claman, E.A. Chaperon, and R.F. Triplett of the School of Medicine at the University of Colorado and A.J.S. Davies of the Chester Beatty Research Institute and Graham F. Mitchell and Jacques Miller of the Walternand Eliza Hall Institute, which demonstrated that in the presence of an antigen the thymic lymphocytes promote the transformation of thymus nondependent lymphocytes in plasma cells.

Collaboration between T lymphocytes leads to the destruction of a virus infected cell. A macrophage that exposes an antigen ingests the virus, digests it, and exposes antigenic viral proteins on the cell membrane together with the class II of MHC molecules. A CD4 lymphocyte is activated when it simultaneously binds the antigen and the protein coded from MHC.

IL-1[5] secreted by the macrophage participates in the activation process. CD4 lymphocyte secretes IL-2 that induces the proliferation of CD8 lymphocytes that have also recognized the antigen together with a MHC class I protein. Some CD8 lymphocytes kill the infected cells that expose the viral antigen, while others depress this cytotoxic response.

CD4 lymphocytes also cooperate with B lymphocytes in the antiviral response. In this case, the interaction with lymphocyte CD4 stimulates the B lymphocyte to proliferate and differentiate into a memory cell clone and a clone of plasma cells secreting antibodies. The antibody molecules bind to the virus by inactivating it. B lymphocytes are also able to recognize the free antigen circulating in the blood and lymph.

In 1970, the cell cooperation was represented as a central element in an "immune orchestra" in which the orchestrals, i.e., B and T lymphocytes and macrophages are directed by a generator of diversity (GOD) (Gershon and Kondo, 1970). In the same year further evidences about the cooperation phenomenon were provided (Mitchison, 1970). In addition, it was demonstrated that antigen recognition participates in both phases, T and B dependent, of the immune response (Raff et al., 1970). Through the possibility of making a compound immunogen by a viral vector conjugation, it was demonstrated that the cooperation occurs through the independent recognition of the vector by helper T lymphocytes and of the hapten by B lymphocytes (Mitchison, 1970; Schirrmacher and Rajewsky, 1970).

A third lymphocyte population is represented by NK (natural killer) cells, characterized by the absence of membrane immunoglobulins or the TCR (T cell receptor). These are lymphocytes with cytotoxic activity in the absence of a previous antigen sensitization (non-MHC restricted cytotoxicity).[6]

Agents of differentiation have been identified, a term coined by Edward A. Boyes and Lloyd J. Old of the New York Research Institute for Sloan Kettering in 1970. For example, the tetra antigen in mice, expressed in both immature and differentiated T cells and but not in B cells. Also in the 1970s, at the National Institute for Medical Research in England, Martin C. Raff was the first to demonstrate that B and T cells can be distinguished from each other through this type of marker.

In 1983, the TCR was discovered and then the TCR coding DNA was isolated which discovered it was constituted by the association of two α and β chains each formed by two independent repetitive domains. The embryonic DNA analysis demonstrated the subdivision in segments called D, D, J whose association are subjected to the same rules of variable parts of antibodies without the presence of mutations. Next, another receptor was described, formed by the association of two γ and δ chains. The complexes formed by the receptors located on the surface of T lymphocytes direct the activity. Both cytotoxic and helper lymphocytes have α-β receptors that can recognize antigens presented on the cell surface by MHC proteins. The coreceptor molecules, also expressed on the surface of cytotoxic and helper lymphocytes, bind to different classes of MHC molecules. When genes encoding for a particular receptor are isolated from a T lymphocyte and inserted into another T lymphocyte provided with a different receptor, it will result in a lymphocyte having both the receptors and able to react against both the antigens recognized by the donor and receiving cell.

The ability to detect TCR is derived from the use of a monoclonal antibody directed to the idiotype of a T lymphocyte to block the antigen response. The identification of this antibody is due to its ability to block a single T lymphocyte clone among many others and from the assumption that the structure responsible for this selectivity corresponds to the combinatory antigen site present on TCR (Haskins et al., 1983). In 1984, Tonegawa and colleagues identified a third gene, the gene γ, which is reassembled by T lymphocytes.

The vast majority of circulating T lymphocytes (more than 90%) includes cells with a α/β TCR, while about 2%–5% of circulating T lymphocytes express a γ/δ TCR. TCRs are expressed in association with a group of proteins forming the so-called CD3 complex. The TCR operates as an antigen recognition element, while the CD3 subunits will act by transducing the activation signal derived from the recognition of the antigen / MHC binomial.

Although TCR and immunoglobulins belong to the same gene superfamily, significant differences between these two receptor types have been found: (1) Ig, unlike TCR, are secreted in significant quantities; (2) Ig recognize soluble antigens, whereas the TCR recognize MHC associated antigens located on the antigen presenting cell membranes;

(3) TCR antigen recognition is facilitated by CD4, accessory molecules expressed on the T cell membrane and interacting with class II MHC molecules expressed on the antigen presenting cells and CD8 interacting with MHC class I molecules; (4) Unlike Ig, TCR does not undergo somatic mutations.

Much of the acquired knowledge about Ig and TCR genes reassortment and other mechanisms that amplify the repertoire of specificity generated by a B or T lymphocyte has been obtained from the study of lymphoproliferative diseases. In contrast, contributions from these basic researches have made it possible to enable the molecular characterization (clonality, differentiation stage, cell line) of leukemia and lymphomas.

## 2.2 THE ROLE OF THE "BURSA OF FABRICIUS" AND THYMUS IN THE IMMUNE RESPONSE

The first description of the bursa of Fabricius was due to Hieronymus Fabricii ("Fabrizio"), born in 1533 in Acquapendente, not far from Rome, and died in Padua in 1619. In 1559 he graduated in Medicine in Padua University where he was a pupil of Gabriele Falloppio, who he replaced as the chair of surgery in 1565. In his work *De formatione ovi et pulli*, he described for the first time the presence of an organ near the cloaca, the "bursa of Fabricius." Fabricii, did not find the bursa in the male bird, so it concluded that its function was a receptacle of semen.[7]

The first evidences of the role of the bursa of Fabricius in the immune response were in the 1950s. In 1954, Bruce Glick, of the Ohio University, was studying the effects of neonatal bursectomy on later chick development and he found that bursectomized chicks grew normally, like the controls. Nine of these chicks were used by one of his collaborators, Chang, during antibody response research, and were treated with the O antigen of *Salmonella typhimurium*. Six animals died immediately after injection; two survived but no antibody response could be highlighted in them. Glick postulated that the early removal of the bursa was responsible for the loss of antibody formation capacity. If the bursa was removed later, the modification of the antibody response was minimal or nothing.

Another technique was used to avoid the development of the bursa. The treatment of embryo with testosterone inhibits the production of antibodies but does not interfere with the ability of animals to reject cutaneous transplants of other animals. Noel L. Warner and Aleksander Szenberg of the Medical Research Institute Walter and Eliza Hall of Melbourne noted in the 1960s that a small number of chicks subjected to this hormonal inhibition tolerated transplants of other animals. However, chicks died immediately after birth, as testosterone exerted negative effects on their development. Warner and Szenberg removed the thymus of these animals, demonstrating a deficiency of lymphocytes and a weak rejection of transplants. Their conclusion was that the thymus and the bursa in the birds have different influences on immunological development.

The B cell precursors start their migration to the bursa epithelium on the 13th day of incubation, 8 days before the birth, and on the 14th day some cells express membrane bound IgM. Some days later is expressed the IgG and before birth the IgA. The bursectomy on 16th−17th development day leads to the absence of all the B cells, resulting in the complete and permanent agammaglobulinemia. When the bursectomy is done on the 19th day, before the birth, IgM are usually present in the adult, while there are no IgG and IgA. When the bursectomy was at birth (21st day), the IgM and IgG are slow to reach normal concentration. In the peripheral lymphoid tissue the sequence of plasma cells development summarizes that of the cells in the bursa; first, synthesized and secreted IgM, then IgG and finally IgA (Moore and Owen, 1966).

In 1961, Jacques F.A.P. Miller of the Chester Beatty Research Institute in London and Robert A. Good of the University of Minnesota, demonstrated that the neonatal mice and rabbits thymectomy was responsible for a severe alteration of cell immunity, consisting of the altered ability of rejection of cutaneous and other tissues transplants. Branislav D. Jankovic, Barry G.W. Arnason, and Byron H. Waksman of the Harvard School of Medicine, demonstrated that the thymus plays a similar role in rats.

The US Immunologist Max D. Cooper noted that also the people with Wiskott−Aldrich syndrome, an X-linked disease, developed viral herpes lesions associated with defective immunity with high levels of antibodies. Conversely, children with agammaglobulinemia were linked to hereditary immunodeficiency of chromosome X control viral infections even though lacking antibody response. He concluded that lymphocytes antibodies producing and the thymus-derived lymphocytes that led to rejection were different from each other.

In 1963, Cooper, Good, and Peterson, at the University of Minnesota, carried out experiments of neonatal bursectomy and thymectomy followed by X-ray exposition, and after irradiation the structure and function of their immune systems were examined. The treated birds were small in size, had fewer lymphocytes, all cellular immune functions were suppressed, and did not produce antibodies.

Irradiated chickens subjected to bursa irradiation, when contaminated with bovine serum albumin or *Brucella abortus* bacteria, did not produce any antibody, although the thymus-dependent internal organs were not affected by the infection. They demonstrated that the bursa influenced the ability to produce antibodies, while does not interfere with the development of cellular immunity. On the other hand, thymectomized animals showed serious cell-mediated immune responses deficiency. Animals subjected to bursectomy and thymectomy had a severe impairment of humoral and cellular immunity.

Using chromosomal markers for tracking the cell precursors migration from bone marrow to thymus and then to spleen and lymph nodes in mice, it was demonstrated that bone marrow included a second lymphocytes population constituted from lymphocytes not passing through the thymus (Ford and Micklem, 1974).

It remained to demonstrate the human equivalent of bursa of Fabricius. In 1974, by the use of fetal liver cell cultures, Cooper, who had moved to London in those years, and some of his colleagues at the University College of London found that these cells originated bone marrow.

At the same time, other researchers made similar findings using bone marrow mice. Hematopoietic tissues, which give rise to all blood cells, are the mammals equivalent of chicken bursa of Fabricius, carrying the same function, or giving rise to B lymphocytes.

The use of specific T and B cell markers permitted the identification of cells involved in lymphatic tumors. Lymphoma induced by aviary viruses is very similar to human Burkitt lymphoma. It seems that the tumor eliciting virus transforms the cells during the clonal differentiation since tumor lymphocytes constantly express IgM. The usual course of gene expression would be interrupted when the cells should pass from the IgM to IgG synthesis.

## 2.3 THE RESOURCE OF NATURAL IMMUNITY AND THE EMERGENCE OF REGULATORY FUNCTION OF CYTOKINES

Natural or innate immunity represents the first line of defense of our organism against pathogens and constitutes the oldest phylogenetic defense mechanism before the development of the specific or adaptive immunity first appeared in vertebrates. In invertebrates, host defense against pathogens is largely mediated by mechanisms of innate immunity. The salient feature of the vertebrate immune system is the expression of antigen binding receptors that have undergone somatic rearrangement as well as most adaptive immune components such as lymphocytes, antibodies and T lymphocyte receptors, MHC molecules, and the presence of specialized lymphoid tissues.

The immune innate mechanisms are preexisting to the microorganism exposition. They include: the epithelial barriers and the antibacterial substances released from epithelial surfaces; phagocytes (neutrophil granulocytes and macrophages); NK cells; the circulating effector proteins, such as the complement, collections and pentraxins; cytokines; chemokines and interferons. Natural immunity cells express receptors (pathogen recognition receptors, PRR) capable of recognizing characteristic structures of microorganisms groups (pathogen-associated molecular patterns). Toll-like receptors (TLR) represent one of the most studied classes of PRR.[8]

By the use of the specific combinations of TLR, the natural immune cells are able to distinguish among the various pathogens classes and then to react directly activating a response able to restrict the pathogen diffusion or stimulating and/or guiding the acquired immune response in the correct direction. TLRs may also be a mechanism for the immune escape of certain pathogenic microorganisms.

The skin and respiratory and intestinal mucosae constitute a physical barrier against the attack of potentially damaging elements. In addition, materials produced by these tissues, such as mucus, contribute to the barrier effect. In the intestine cavity, mucus creates a "fluid barrier" that slows down the passage of the bacteria, facilitating recognition and possibly destruction by the defense mechanisms.

If the microorganisms overcome the epithelial barriers they encounter macrophages that phagocytize the pathogen to digest it. Phagocytes are not limited to removing molecules, virus, and bacteria from tissues, but they also deal with transforming their components into substances that are not able to damage the tissues. Macrophages do not only deal with the organism resistance against aggressive external agents but are involved in the elimination of metabolic components to prevent their accumulation to excess.

At the same time the macrophages release cytokines[9] which promote the recruitment of blood stream lymphocytes such as the neutrophils to the inflammation site. Macrophages are phylogenetically the oldest innate immune cells. *Drosophila* responds to infections by "hemocytes," very similar to macrophages.

It was around the 1970s that the role of cytokines began to take shape, with the identification of molecules participating in the immune system communication network, produced by the same immune system cells but different from the antibodies. Cytokines action is fundamentally local (autocrine or paracrine) and their secretion is mostly a short duration and self-limiting phenomenon. They are generally ex novo produced, following stimulation, through the transcription of specific genes, and are never accumulated as preformed molecules in the cell. Cytokine receptors are membrane glycoproteins formed by different subunits and, depending on the structural homology among extracellular domains, are grouped into multiple families; each receptor family is different from the other, and each member within a family is a protein variant with its own structural characteristics, capable of inducing a specific function in the cell that exposes it.

The innate response against viruses is based on the production of interferons which are antiviral cytokines and on the activation of NK cells which kill the virus infected cells. The Italian immunologist Lorenzo Moretta, with his team in Genoa, over the last 20 years, has discovered how and why NK cells are capable of blocking leukemic or virus-infected cells and not most normal cells. In particular Moretta discovered new inhibitory receptors specific for class I HLA molecules (termed Kir) and receptors responsible for the NK cells activation and the induction of tumor cell death processes. Genes coding for these receptors were cloned in his laboratory in Genoa. Overall, over 15 new receptor molecules have been identified and cloned. The knowledge acquired on NK cells and their receptors are the bases of important results in acute high risk leukemia based on the identification of *mismatches* between donor NK cell KIR receptors and patient class I alleles (typically, in haploidentical parent transplant, or partially compatible donor).

Pathogens capable of resisting these defense mechanisms enter into blood circulation, where they are recognized by innate immunity proteins, as the complement system.

Chemokines are small polypeptide cytokines produced by macrophages, endothelial cells, and various other cytotypes in response to microbial products and to IL-1 and tumor necrosis factor (TNF).[10]

Pentraxins are a group of pentameric proteins including the short pentraxins such as the reactive C protein and serum amylod P protein and the long pentraxin PTX3. PTX3 was discovered by the Italian immunologist Alberto Mantovani in Milan in the early 1990s. From that moment Mantovani began to study every aspect of PTX3: from its first application in diagnosis to the discovery of its role during the infections against *Aspergillus fumigatus* bacterium, to its role in immune response. In 2010 the gene was cloned and its structure was analyzed. Studies that led to the understanding that PTX3 carries out its function at the inflammatory stage by interacting with another protein, P-selectin, expressed by endothelial cells in the presence of tissue damage or inflammatory stimulation. By the interaction with P-selectin, PTX3 slows down and limits the leukocytes infiltration in the inflammatory site, acting locally to reduce their recruitment and so regulating the inflammatory response. More recently, the role of PTX3 as an oncosuppressor has been highlighted.

The renewed interest in the innate immunity mechanisms is documented by the Nobel Prize awarded to Bruce Beutler, Professor of Genetics and Immunology at the Scripps Research Institute in La Jolla, California, together with the French Immunologist Jules Hoffman (1941) of the University of Strasbourg and the Canadian biologist Ralph Steinman (1943–2011).

The researches carried out by Beutler permitted to better understand the functioning mechanism of the immune system, clarifying the defense mechanisms against foreign agents such as viruses and bacteria. Such studies are also offering important results for the development of vaccines able to guide the immune system in attacking tumor cells and in general for the design of new treatment strategies for inflammatory and autoimmune diseases.

The discovery of the genetic mechanism that causes and controls the innate immune response in insects was made by Jules Hoffmann and it is included in a series of extremely brilliant studies that have followed since the late 1980s. The publication in "Cell" in 1996 showed that the coding gene of a membrane receptor called *toll* (already known for its role in the development of *Drosophila*) was crucial in triggering the defense of the insect against a mycotic infection was one of the decisive steps. The genes involved in the cascade leading from *toll* receptor to the production of antimycotic and antibacterial peptides (for Gram-positive bacteria) as well as defense mechanisms against Gram-negative bacteria were subsequently identified by a group of researchers in Strasbourg. These discoveries were followed by TLR receptors in mammals, homologous of the *toll* insect receptor.

Professor Beutler was the first to clone, in 1998, the gene of one of these TLR in which the binder is a bacterial lipopolysaccharide (LPS) also called endotoxin, which is responsible for septic shock. In total, 13TLR were subsequently identified among mammals. They are expressed in particular by dendritic cells, B lymphocytes, as well as numerous other cell types. Each of them has specificity for an antigenic substance or a group of them: TLR4 recognizes LPS, others bind to nucleic acids (TLR3, TLR7, TLR8, and TLR9), one to lipoproteins and glycolipids (TLR2), flagellin (bacterial flagellate component) (TLR5), and so on. The TLR are therefore essential sensors in the interactions between the organism and its environment. These discoveries have given rise to clinical applications. Much work on TLR has been conducted in order to increase, modulate, or inhibit inflammatory reactions in different circumstances: e.g., in order to better design vaccines, mitigate allergic phenomena and autoimmune reactions, or correct immunodeficiencies. In addition to these contributions, Bruce Beutler isolated TNF and discovered its very important role in inflammatory processes. TNF blocking activity agents are now widely used in medical practice to inhibit the progression of many autoimmune diseases.

Ralph Steinman, professor of immunology at Rockefeller University, New York, discovered dendritic cells in 1973. Unfortunately, the scientist died 3 days before receiving the Nobel Prize[11]. Dendritic cells are cells specialized in the antigen capture and presentation and constitute the conjunction ring between innate and adaptive immunity. In tissues they play an immune system sentinel role and are able to detect the presence of microbes by specific receptors. The interaction of the pathogen with these receptors induces its internalization, which may equally occur by macropinocytosis in dendritic cells. In addition, dendritic cells carry antigens to secondary lymphoid organs and present them to T lymphocytes.

## ENDNOTES

1. In 1901, Metchnikoff wrote: "Macrophages preferably take possession of animal cells, such as blood globules, spermatozoa and all other animal deriving elements. Among infectious microorganisms, macrophages have a predilection for those who cause chronic diseases such as leprosy, tuberculosis and actinomycosis and also those that reveal an animal nature. In this latter category are amoeboid parasites of malaria, Texas fever, and trypanosomes are included. Macrophages can also incorporate acute diseases bacteria, but exceptionally, their intervention is of little importance" (*Immunization in Infectious Diseases*, Corbellini, 1990, p. 95).

2. Interferons are a family of natural proteins correlated to each other. They were discovered in 1957 at the National Institute of Medical Research of London when Scottish virologist Alick Isaacs and Swiss physician Jean Lindermann identified a new antiviral protein. They termed it interferon because it seemed it was the agent of viral interference. Since the 1930s, it has been shown that infection with a virus interferes for a certain period of time with infection by other viruses. Isaacs and Lindermann found that the first virus not only blocked the access of other viruses into the same cells, but also induced in the infected cells the release of something into the culture medium. When the media was added to another cell culture the latter became resistant to the virus. Interferons are classified into three major groups ($\alpha$, $\beta$, and $\gamma$) based on cell origin and their induction agents and historically have been studied for their antiviral activity. After binding to specific receptors, they induce the activation of signal transduction pathways that stimulate a wide range of genes that have not only antiviral but also immunomodulatory and antiproliferative activity. The inhibition of viral growth and/or cell proliferation by interferons is associated with various physiological changes, some of which depend on the activity of specific proteins that are interferon-inducible.

3. By acronym IL-1 is defined a proteins family composed by IL-1$\alpha$ and IL-1$\beta$ with pleiotropic activity, involved in immune and inflammatory responses during the infections. The biochemical studies carried out in the 1970s have shown that the IL-1 is mainly produced by macrophages.

4. The lymphocytes possess the so-called "cluster of differentiation" membrane antigen. This term was introduced for the first time in 1982 at the first Conference on Leukocyte Differentiation Antigens, with the aim of classifying the different monoclonal antibodies.

5.  In 1974, a product called the lymphocyte activating factor (LAF) corresponding to IL-1 able to induce the proliferation of mouse thymocytes, was identified in the supernatants of activated human leukocytes. IL-1 biological activities are various: it stimulates the proliferation and differentiation of T cells; it plays an important role in activating B lymphocytes, in the fibroblasts proliferation, and in stimulating the synthesis of inflammatory proteins; acts synergically with hematopoietic growth factors on highly immature bone marrow precursors; induces the production of IL-2 which in turn stimulates the proliferation of T lymphocytes (Gershon et al., 1974).

6.  In 1988 the NK cell international workshop identified them as large granular lymphocytes (LGL), great lymphocytes with high nucleus/cytoplasm ratio, indented nucleus containing azurophilic granules. These cells, representing 15% of the lymphocytes present in the blood, do not express CD3 on their surface, or one of the TCR chains, express CD16 and mediate cytolytic reactions in the absence of class I or II MHC molecules on target cells. These cells were discovered in the United States in the mid-1960s by Ron Herberman and in Sweden by Eva Klein. In Italy, the contribution to their characterization by Lorenzo and Alessandro Moretta and Carlo E. Grossi, immunologists working in Genoa, was fundamental.

7.  Girolamo Fabrizi d'Acquapendente, in addition to being the founder of an important School of Practice Medicine in Padua, was particularly distinguished for the embryology and physiology studies. The inauguration of the new anatomical theater in Padua in 1594 was due to Fabrizi, designed by Paolo Sarpi. Fabrizi, in his university lessons, compared human and animal anatomy. Fabrizi considered the egg growth and was the first to understand that the ovary and the oviduct play a crucial role in the formation and nourishment of the egg. Then he discussed the structure, function, and utility of different types of eggs and later the formation, growth, and nutrition of the chick. He adopted the Aristotle interpretation according to which it was the female who provided all matter and the male the shape, to conclude that the cock's semen was stored in the cloacal bursa (the "Fabricius bursa"), while the eel at the base of the egg was the matter by which the chick takes shape.

8.  Named after the recognizing of the TOLL receptor in Drosophila, *Toll-like* receptors or TLR represent the main class of innate immunity receptors. They have been identified eleven until now in humans, numbered from TLR1 to TLR11. Structurally they are transmembrane proteins that have a common extracellular domain that consists of a series of rich in leucine and cysteine replications and an intracellular domain that plays a primary role in signal transduction. Various TLRs recognize several microbial components, including LPS peptidoglycans, non-methylated c-phosphate-c CpG nucleotides (all molecules present predominantly in microorganisms), single and double helix RNA. These receptors, once activated, stimulate the production of bactericidal substances.

9.  In relation to their mainly carried out function, the different cytokines can be distinguished in: mediators of immunity; mediators of inflammatory response; regulators of differentiation and cell growth; growth factors.

10. Chemokines represent a large family of structurally homologous cytokines that can stimulate leukocyte movement by leading the migration from blood stream to tissues. About 50 chemokines have been identified in humans, all structurally similar to each other. These can be grouped into four subfamilies based on the number and position of the N-terminal cysteine residues responsible for disulphide bridges: (1) the chemokines CC, wherein the first two sulphide bridges are adjacent; (2) the CXC chemokines, wherein the same residues are separated from an amino acid; (3) chemokines C, which possess only one cysteine residue; (4) and CX3C chemokines, which have two cysteine residues separated by three amino acids.

11. The unexpected news raised a problem: according to the letter of the Nobel Foundation regulations, the award cannot be conferred on memory, unless the death of the honored person occurs between the date of the announcement (in October) and the award ceremony (the December 10). After a reexamination the problem, the Committee reaffirmed the award of the prize to Steinman with the following reasoning: "The interpretation of the purpose of this rule leads to the conclusion that Ralph Steinman will be awarded the 2011 Nobel Prize for Physiology or Medicine. The purpose of the abovementioned rule is to clarify that Nobel Prize cannot be deliberately assigned posthumously. However, the decision to award the Nobel Prize to Ralph Steinman was taken in good faith, based on the assumption that the Nobel Prize was alive. The Nobel Foundation therefore believes that what has occurred recalls rather than the case provided by the statute for a person who has been marked as Nobel Prize and died before the award ceremony. The decision taken by the Nobel Assembly of the Karolinska Institutet therefore remains unchanged."

# CHAPTER 3

# The Genetic Basis of Immune Response

## 3.1 ANTIGEN RECOGNITION CONTROLLED BY MAJOR HISTOCOMPATIBILITY COMPLEX

In 1936 Peter Gorer was the first to identify the major histocompatibility complex (MHC) as a crucial locus during the transplantation reject processes called *histocompatibility*-2 (H-2) in inbred mice (genetically equal to each other).

At the end of the 1960s the physiological function of MHC molecules was demonstrated by Baruch Benaceraff of New York University and Hugh O. McDevitt, who had previously worked in Israel and then at Harvard University. These researchers showed that certain guinea pig and mouse strains synthesized antibodies against certain protein antigens while others were unable. McDevitt demonstrated that responsiveness depended on particular type of MHC class II molecules expressed by mice (H-2).

It was thus possible to establish that MHC is a gene complex formed by multiple and polymorphic loci that encode for histocompatibility molecules. The expression of these molecules (MHC antigens) on cell surfaces generates an individual genetic diversity responsible for the transplant rejection phenomenon. According to Hilliard Festenstein of London Hospital Medical College this gene complex would have been highly conserved during evolution in various animal species.

In the 1940s, US biologist George D. Snell (1903−96, Nobel Prize in 1980), with French immunologist Jean Dausset (1916−2009), and Baruj Benacerraf (1920−2011), an American national Venezuelan physiologist, created by particular crossbreeds a mice strain identical for all genome traits, except the loci or gene region coding for the histocompatibility antigens. In this way, it was possible to identify and localize the different loci at gene level and to demonstrate the allelic variability with serological methods. In 1950, Dausset, in the meantime he was working in Paris, isolated the first antibodies in multitransfused

Immunology in the Twentieth Century. DOI: https://doi.org/10.1016/B978-0-12-816145-6.00003-2

patients, which made it possible to highlight the close analogy between the mouse H-2 molecules and HLA (human leukocyte antigens, so-called because they used leukocytes for donors and recipients in transplants typization) encoded by human MHC, providing an important instrument of defining individual antigens of HLA. The HLA system includes a set of genes located on chromosome n.6. The exact location of the genome region results from studies performed on hamster/man somatic hybrids, in which it was observed that some markers, already located on chromosome n.6, and the HLA antigens segregated with the same chromosome. Dausset discovered that the serum of the people who had received numerous transfusions tended to react in the presence of white bodies of other individuals causing the agglutination. The Italian Ruggero Ceppellini[1] gave a fundamental contribution to the characterization of the HLA system.

In parallel to Dausset, Rose Payne at Stantford and Jan Van Rood at Leida independently discovered that serum from mothers who had more children could induce the white blood cells of other people to agglutinate themselves. Van Rood gained her insight from the severe reaction that occurred to a mother as a consequence of a single transfusion and assumed that the woman had been sensitized during her previous pregnancy by the nonself-proteins derived by the father of the children. She came in contact with the blood or cells of each child during the delivery.

Next, they defined the functions and the allelic (nucleotidic) variability of the loci coding for the two main classes of membrane molecules, the class I histocompatibility molecules expressed on the exogenous antigen presenting cells. In humans, the HLA system includes three loci of class I (A, B, and C) and three of class II (DR, DP, and DQ). In addition, each locus of class II includes genes A and B that respectively encode the A and B chains of a single molecule of class II. The different alleles of these genes that we can inherit by our parents are very similar to each other but they have subtle differences that have been cataloged. When an individual is exposed or transplanted by cells or tissues of a genetically different donor (allogenic) the recipient produces antibodies reacting against antigens codified by HLA loci.

Since 1964 a decisive role in this research area has been carried out by a close collaboration among the researchers through the material and methodologies exchanges and the organization of biennial international workshops. The research has been developed on three main directives: a more precise knowledge of the genetic and molecular structure of HLA-A, -B, and -C loci and their corresponding genes; the identification of serologically definable specificities related to D antigens; the localization in the HLA region of loci not involved or only partially involved in the histocompatibility.

The biological significance of the HLA chromosome region arises by the examination of the literature regarding the association between particular HLA antigens and the diseases. It regards pathologies that have been shown to be clearly familiar, with a subacute or chronic progression, which rarely influence survival during the fertile age; they are therefore diseases having little impact on reproduction and so do not have great effect on the survival of the species. The most significant association regards the B27 HLA and ankylosing spondylitis in which approximately 96% of patients possess this particular allele. Another antigen frequently associated to autoimmune pathogenesis diseases (celiac disease, myasthenia severe, herpetic dermatitis) is the B8.

The first demonstration that MHC molecules represent an antigen recognition system was due to Hugh O. McDevitt, who worked at the National Institute of Medical Research in London, and Bauj Benacerraf, who worked at Harvard. The two researchers demonstrated that genes located in MHC can control the immune response against different synthetic antigens. These genes—indicated as immune response genes or Ir genes—were subsequently identified with the genes coding for class II histocompatibility antigens. An animal possessing a variant of a particular gene of the MHC complex could begin a very effective response against an antigen, while another animal that has a different variant might not give any response.

With regards to the MHC system, in 1981 Benacerraf, wrote:

*As concerns the individual sphere, the existence of such a polymorphic system that controls specific responsiveness and suppression will inevitably create individuals different to each other in their immunological potential response against an antigenic challenge. Some of them clearly will be at greater risk, while others will result as better prepared to resist to certain infectious agents, and it is no surprise that immunologic diseases are linked to MHC. Thus, as concerns the species, this defense system represents a very important selective advantage during the unpredictable response and a better chance for the immune system to adapt to evolutionary pressures. (The role of MHC gene products in the regulation of immune function, in Corbellini, 1990, p. 294)*

In 1974, a physician from Basel, Rolf Martin Zinkernagel, and an Australian neuropathologist Peter Charles Doherty (Nobel Prize in 1996), working at the John Curtin School of Medical Research in Camberra, Australia, showed that certain mouse strains died as a consequence of a cerebral infection caused by lymphocytic coriomeningitis virus. These mice, in response to the viruses, produced cytotoxic T lymphocytes expressing a particular group of class I MHC molecules that attacked the infected nervous system. The lytic effect occurred only in the presence of a MHC identity between the effector cells and the target; the T cell had to recognize two signals on the target: the antigen and the MHC. The two researchers found that if the class I MHC proteins located on the surface of these new infected cells differed from those of the original mouse, these new cells escaped the action of T lymphocytes and also demonstrated that the isolated T mouse lymphocytes were able to recognize cells infected with a second animal virus only if both the animals expressed the same class I molecules. Finally, Zinkernagel and Doherty demonstrated that cellular interactions were subjected to genetic restriction imposed by H-2 complex products.

In the next 10 years, Emil R. Unanue, first at Harvard and then at Washington University, and Howard M. Gray, at Denver's National Jewish Center for Immunology and Respiratory Medicine, showed that to stimulate an immune response, extracellular proteins must first be endocyted and fragmented into peptides by an antigen presenting cell. The peptides thus bind to class II MHC molecules that are expressed on the cell surface as a complex that can be recognized by T helper lymphocytes.

## 3.2 IMMUNOGENETIC

In 1901, Landsteiner mixed up all the possible combinations of serum and red blood cells of 22 donors from his laboratory and observed that some sera induced the agglutination of red blood cells of other patients but not their own. He had discovered the A, B, zero blood groups system. By these experiments Landsteiner expressed some conclusions: in the human red blood cells there were two antigenic determinants which he defined as A and B. Some persons possessed the A antigen and were members of group A; others, on the other hand, possessed the B one and were members of the group B. There was a third group called the group zero, composed of persons in which there were neither of the two antigens. Next, it was demonstrated that the members of the group zero expressed the H heterogeneous antigen.

Furthermore, the Landsteiner work demonstrated that all the individuals possess a type of antibodies in the sera, the so-called naturally produced isoagglutinins directed against antigenic determinants not contained in their erythrocytes. Thus individuals in group A possess anti-B antibodies, and individuals in group B possess anti-A antibodies. Individuals of the zero group possess anti-A and anti-B antibodies and individuals in the AB group do not possess anti-A or anti-B antibodies. When Landsteiner illustrated the results of his experiments he said, "I hope this discovery will be of some use."

In 1939, a study was conducted in a newborn affected by a severe form of hemolytic disease, characterized by intense jaundice, generalized edema, and hepatosplenomegaly, which was termed fetal erythroblastosis. After the delivery, the mother of this newborn was affected by an intense reaction following a blood transfusion by her husband (Levine and Stetson, 1939).

In 1940, Landsteiner and the US immunologist Alexander Wiener (1907–76) immunized rabbits through the *Macacus rhesus* monkey red blood cells, with the intent of demonstrating the possible existence of new human isoantigens, and discovered that the antibodies produced could induce agglutination in 85% of the erythrocytes population, but not in the remaining 15%.

These observations led to the discovery of a new antigenic determinant which was called Rho factor, which indicated the species of *Rhesus* erythrocytes used in the experimental antibodies production.

Moreover, the clinical case was explained as the acquisition of a paternal isoantigen, extraneous to the mother one, by the fetus erythrocytes when passed into the mother's circle giving rise to an isoimmunization. The antibodies were transferred from the mother to the fetus causing the hemolytic reaction. The discovery of Landsteiner and Weiner constituted a fundamental stage for the study of maternal–fetal immunological relationships.

Immunogenetics was born, whose field of investigation ranges from the population genetic study through the use of antigenic markers to immune response genetic control analysis.

## 3.3 IMMUNE TOLERANCE AND THE IMMUNOLOGICAL BASIS OF TRANSPLANT REJECTION

Immune tolerance can be defined as the inability to give rise to a specific immune response to a given antigen, as a consequence of the previous exposure to the same antigen.

In 1945, Ray Owen, who worked at Wisconsin University in the United States, was studying the blood groups of nonidentical twin calves (dizygotes). He observed that each twin possessed, in addition to their own red blood cells, also red blood cells with antigens corresponding to the genetic heritage of the other twin.

Each twin was also able to accept skin grafts from the other twin, but not from genetically unrelated calves. Since the dizygous calves in intrauterine life share the same placental circulation, it was believed that the phenomenon was due to the mutual exchange of red blood cells of their progenitors and that the failure in the elimination of allogeneic cells was related to the cellular exchange occurred when the immune system was not completely mature.

As Tauber wrote (1999, p. 77): "Although the 'self-configuration' is inherited, the recognition of its components takes place during development. Therefore, these markers represent the basis of the discrimination between the self and not, allowing this recognition to inhibit an immune response where it appears inappropriate."

Burnet was influenced by Owen's work and interpreted the tolerance observed in identical twins as a form of hyporeactivity. He hypothesized that it must have developed in the calves when they entered in contact with each other's cells during the fetal stage, and so he developed with Frank Fenner the concept of an self-marker, acquired during the early stages of life, whose presence prevented the self body components from participating in the immune processes.

According to Burnet and Fenner (1948, p. 38):

*Among the cells potentially producing antibodies there are enzymatic groups generally adapted to 'correspond' to a enough number of marker components to allow the differentiation of the self by the organic foreign material (i.e., the normal invasive microorganisms). When this 'correspondence' occurs, normal disintegration processes happen without stimulating immune activity. An antigen is such by virtue of fact that, due to its general chemical characteristics, it corresponds to one or the other of the self-markers, but it will adapt to the corresponding enzyme only when it is deformed in an appropriate adaptive configuration. This aforementioned deformation provides the stimulus for the replication and the release of antibodies.*

In the early 1930s, it was observed that skin grafts between members of the same family tend to survive longer than those between unrelated individuals (Padget, 1932).

A few years later it was demonstrated that the monozygotic twins (genetically identical) could accept skin grafts from each other (Brown, 1937).

Crucial research was conducted by the Scottish surgeon Tom Gibson and the British biologist and zoologist Peter B. Medawar (1915–1987) at the Burns Department of the Glasgow Royal Infirmary during the Second World War where they treated burns in aviators. The skin grafts were indispensable for the extended burns treatment.[2] The two researchers demonstrated that a second graft from another donor was rejected more rapidly than the first.

When Medawar came back to Oxford, he executed skin grafts on rabbits confirming that the skin cannot be permanently transplanted from a rabbit to another genetically different from the first. Each graft survived only some weeks. When the transplant was repeated the second time the reject was more rapid than the first and if the graft belonged to a rabbit different from the first skin donor, the reject occurred slowly. If as an alternative it derived by the same first donor, the reject occurred more rapidly (Medawar, 1944, 1945).

In 1947, Medawar became professor of Zoology at the Birmingham University and in 1951 he moved to the University College of London. Here he carried out a series of experiments that led him to publish in collaboration with the English biologist Rupert E. Billingham (1921–2002) and the immunologist Leslie Brent (1925) a crucial work in "Nature" in 1953. Through the inspiration derived from Owen's work they demonstrated that when inbred pups mice belonging to genetically pure A strain were injected with bone marrow or spleen derived cells collected by mice belonging to a different genetically not related cba strain, it made the animals belonging to A strain permissive towards the allogenic transplanted cells and able to accept a skin graft belonging to animals of strain cba but not from animals of another strain.

The results of this work were supplemented by other data included in a new work published in 1956. After Billingham's departure for America, Brent and Medawar focused their attention on the inducing tolerance theory in adult animals and on the relationships between reactivity to homotransplants and delayed hypersensitivity reactions, considering the sensitized lymphocyte instead of the antibodies as agents of the immune response.

In 1960, Medawar and Burnet received the Nobel Prize for Medicine. Medawar recognized the important role carried out by Billingham and Brent with whom he wanted to share the cash prize. Furthermore, Medawar also wrote to Owen believing it to be unfair that the award had not been also attributed to him, when he had been the initiator of this research field.

The tolerance can also be determined by soluble antigens. For example, the administration of bovine serum albumin without any adjuvant in rabbits after birth prevents the antibodies production as response to this protein. To maintain tolerance the antigen needs to persist in the individual. In the Medawar experiments the tolerance status continued because the animals were chimeric, possessing both the A and CBA cells. The tolerance is gradually lost when soluble antigens such as the albumin were used. This could occur because when the antigen is absent there is a new recruitment of immunocompetent cells before they turn into tolerant. Also for this reason the tolerance status persists more in timectomized animals.

In 1954 the surgeon Joseph Murray (1919–2012), of the Peter Bent Brigham Hospital in Boston, executed a kidney transplant between dizygotic or monovular twins (the organs of which were indistinguishable to their respective immune systems) using sublethal X-ray.

In 1960, the immunosuppressive effects of the antimitotic drug 6-mercaptopurine (Schwartz and Dameshek, 1960) were demonstrated and in 1962 Murray was able to transplant an unrelated cadaveric kidney, under the azathioprine, derived from 6-mercaptopurine, immunosuppressive protection. Since the 1980s, ciclosporin, discovered in 1969, has further improved the possibility of post-transplant survival. Since then the evolution of medical practice has made relatively simple and common the transplantations of heart, liver, and pancreas.

In 1990, the Nobel Prize was conferred to Murray and to the American physician Edward Donnall Thomas (1920–2012), who together with Robert Good and the American oncologist Georges W. Santos (1928–2001), had executed the transplantation of allogeneic hematopoietic stem cells, between the end of the 1960s to the early 1970s. The recipient was irradiated with lethal doses to destroy the malignant cells (in the case of leukemias) or to create a possibility of implantation (in the case of aplastic anemias). In Italy, the hematopoietic stem cells transplantation pioneers were Alberto Marmont from Genoa, Glauco Torlontano from Pescara, and Guido Lucarelli from Pesaro.[3]

In 1957, a different syngeneic or allogenic stem cells transplantation subjected animals survival was reported (Barnes and Loutit, 1957).[4] In the same year it was observed that severe diarrhea, weight loss, and skin lesions appeared as a secondary disease in mice transplanted with allogeneic splenic cells (Van Bekkum and Vos, 1957). Next, it became clear that what were responsible for this phenomenon were lymphocytes, with the lymphatic system, liver, skin, and gut as principal targets.

During the 1970s, the transplantation reject phenomenon was analyzed in vitro by Terry Brunner and Jean-Charles Cerottini who evaluated the T helper lymphocyte proliferative response against allogenic histocompatibility antigens (expressed in cells of different individuals of the same species) and the generation of cytotoxic T lymphocytes capable of killing allogenic and tumor target cells.

In the mid-1960s, Billingham defined the characteristics of the so-called graft versus host disease (GVHD) through the use of both animal and human models: the donor's cells must be immunologically competent; the host has to contain some crucial antigens that are not present in the donor that make him appear as foreign; the host is unable to organize an immunological reaction against transplantation. GVHD was defined as a consequence of the synergism between the immunological damage due to the HLA system antigenic incompatibility and the tissue damage caused by irradiation or viral infections. In the GVHD, the immunocompetent T cells of the donor recognize the recipient's tissue as foreign and react against it, damaging it.

# ENDNOTES

1. Ceppellini, who had completed the medical studies at the end of Second World War, worked at the Blood Bank and at the Immunology Laboratory of the University of Milan until 1952, and then he was called to the Institute of Genetics of the University of Turin. Since the 1960 he was part of an immunologist group installed by the World Health Organization to rewrite the immunoglobulins nomenclature. In 1967, he introduced the haplotype concept in order to define the group of genetic determinants that are inherited by one of the parents. His studies on the transplant immunology were fundamental. He has been repeatedly nominated for the Nobel Prize.

2. Medawar developed a method for separation of the epidermis from the dermis by trypsin treatment, and attempted to cover the burned areas with suspensions of epidermal cells. The application of this method did not give any positive results because it did not stop the destructive process of wound retraction.

3. Transplant for genetic diseases, especially for thalassemia major has had particular development in Italy. After the first transplant carried out in Seattle on a 2-year-old Italian child who was not transfused because he was a son of Jehovah's Witnesses, thousands of transplants were performed, the vast majority in Italy. Pioneers in this field were the Pesaro group, led by Lucarelli, and Pescara group, led by Torlontano. The Italian experience has demonstrated that by hematopoietic stem cell transplantation it is possible to obtain a permanent correction of anemia in thalassemia subjects with a follow-up of over 20 years.

4. Bone marrow transplantation refers to the infusion of hematopoietic stem cells derived by the same individual or a donor into an individual. The first case is called autologous transplantation, the second one is the allogenic transplant. Stem cells are obtained from bone marrow, peripheral blood, or umbilical cord blood.

# CHAPTER 4

# Immune System Pathologies

## 4.1 IMMUNE DISORDERS

The evolution of pathogenetic knowledge about immunodeficiencies is closely linked to the definition of ontogenesis and the anatomical–functional organization of the immune system. Furthermore, the development of immunoelectrophoresis techniques has allowed a more precise definition of Ig defects of many conditions in which hypogammaglobulinemia affects one or two classes of Ig, while levels of other classes are normal or increased.

In 1950, there was a report of the case of two unrelated children who died of sepsis during the second year of life after suffering from continuous and serious infections represented by lung diseases, diarrhea, thrush, and persistent morbilliform rash. Since in both cases it had occurred with a severe lymphopenia, this disease was called "essential lymphocytosis" (Glanzmann and Riniker, 1950).

The first clinical case description of antibody immune response deficiency was published in 1952 in "Pediatrics" by Colonel Ogden Bruton, a primary physician at the Walter Reed Army Center. It was an 8-year-old child with a history of recurrent episodes of pneumococcal sepsis, such as pneumonia, purulent otitis media, and septic arthritis, which had lasted 4 years and whose serum electrophoretic pattern lacked the γ peak. Before proceeding with the electrophoretic analysis, there had been made attempts to control recurrent infections with chemo-, serum-, and vaccine therapy. At that time the medical literature had described cases of hypoproteinemia due to nephrosis or hyponutrition. Bruton also had the merit of trying for the first time the substitutive treatment with gammaglobulins that led to the child's clear improvement and he could have a normal growth in the following years.

Bruton pointed out in his article that the patient was not affected by nephrotic syndrome and that he fed normally. According to

Immunology in the Twentieth Century. DOI: https://doi.org/10.1016/B978-0-12-816145-6.00004-4

Bruton, the clinical picture could be attributed either to a congenital or acquired deficiency of the antibody production mechanism. In fact, the case described by Bruton was not a congenital sex-linked agamma-globulinemia or Bruton type because the histological examination of the tonsils, bone marrow, and liver showed that the structure of these organs was normal.

The Bruton disease or X-recessive agammaglobulinemia (xla or X-linked agammaglobulinemia) consists of an acquired X-linked immunodeficiency, characterized by the inability of the affected people to produce Ig and therefore antibodies. It depends on a chromosome X associated gene mutation encoding the Bruton tyrosine kinase (BTK) and it is characterized by a defect of B lymphocytes maturation. Individuals affected by this immunodeficiency have pre-B cells with normal μ chains, but, due to the lack of tyrosine kinase function, the subsequent light chains genes rearrangement process does not occur, thus the pre-B lymphocytes do not mature to B lymphocytes.

The children affected by Bruton type-agammaglobulinemia rarely get sick during the first 6 months of life, because they are covered by antibodies received from the mother. The agammaglobulinemia syn-drome case picture was characterized by serious recurrent infections (pneumonia, meningitis, sepsis, otitis, synovitis, and conjunctivitis) associated with a circulating gamma globulin marked deficiency. These children exceeded the mycotic infections and most viral infections with relative ease, instead going to meet very serious, often deadly, morbid manifestations as a result of infections by pyogenic germs. Bruton also demonstrated that the administration of the plasma fraction character-ized by IgG antibodies in the same patient resulted in a significant reduction in recurrent infections.

According to Good, "when antibiotics were not yet available the patients affected by this dysfunction succumbed to the first or one of the first bacterial infections. Thus the sequence of infections that now char-acterized the syndrome was not observed" (Good et al., 1962, p. 252).

In 1952, three types of agammaglobulinemia were detected: (a) *congenital*, observed in male children and characterized by recurrent bacterial infections occurring in childhood or at the time of early puberty; (b) *acquired*, observed in individual belonging to both sexes, in whom a series of serious recurrent infections could occur starting from puberty throughout life; (c) *transient*, observed in early infancy, from the 6th to 9th month of life and which spontaneously regresses around 3 years, as a consequence of a defect in the autonomous synthesis of antibodies by the infant, which in the first months of life after birth is defended by Ig of maternal origin (Gitlin and Janeway, 1956).

In the same year it was also demonstrated that plasma cells were not present in the bone marrow of agammaglobulinemic patients and that antibodies were not synthesized in these patients following antigenic stimulation. Moreover, the lymph node germinal centers were absent and the tonsils hypotrophic. On the other hand, the T-dependent paracortical areas of the lymph nodes were normally developed and atrophic following antigenic stimulation (Good and Zack, 1956). Finally, in the same year the case of a patient with a thymoma was described that in addition to low antibodies levels showed a reduced ability to reject allografts and to elaborate a delayed hypersensitivity response (Good et al., 1956).

In 1968, Angelo M. Di George, a pediatrician at Temple University's School of Medicine, discovered that the children born without thymus presented few circulating lymphocytes and lacked immune cell functions, without any alteration of circulating antibodies and plasma cells, and showed an abnormal susceptibility to viral and fungal infections. In children affected by this pathology did not develop epithelial anlagen derived from the third and fourth branchial pouches, which give rise to the thymus during embryonic development. Also the cells arising from neural crest contribute to the thymic epithelial anlagen formation and the lacking of their migration leads to a defect in the thymus development and reduction of T lymphocytes. From the third branchial pouch originates also the mandible, the two superior parathyroids, the cone and the trunk of pulmonary artery, and the origin of aorta. Thus, in the George syndrome there are a variable combination of defects in the development of parathyroids, the thymus, the arterial cone of the pulmonary artery, the ascending aorta and the aortic arch, and craniofacial anomalies.

Children generally arrive at pediatric observation following an attack of neonatal tetany due to parathyroid insufficiency. Children with thymic aplasia who survive the neonatal period have a tendency to contract infections from viruses, fungi, and bacteria that can be very serious. The clinical syndrome features are extremely heterogeneous; in the classical form they include neonatal hypocalcemic tetany, immuno-deficiency of the cellular immunity, congenital cardiopathies, thymus aplasia, and facial dysmorphia. This phenotype, over time, has been extended also to patients who presented only some of the classic symptoms. Congenital cardiopathies are present in 75% of affected individuals and are the main cause of morbidity and mortality and often the first symptom during the neonatal period. In 1968, a human fetal thymus was transplanted into a patient affected by Di George syndrome followed by a rapid restoring of immunological functions (Cleveland et al., 1968).

Immune deficiency syndromes are divided into primary and secondary forms. The primary ones represent the real immune deficiency pathologies with a genetic basis and appear in the pediatric or often neonatal age. In this group a subgroup of late primary, or acquired, forms of the adult can be considered. In primitive immune deficiencies the risk of developing a lymphoma is about 10 to 200 times higher than in the normal population and lesions usually occur in young individuals.

The secondary forms concern immune deficiencies associated to another disease that differently from the primary forms, affect the immune response in a complete developed immune system. It is known that patients with Hodgkin disease[1] are particularly exposed to the tuberculosis, fungal, and viral infections.[2] Multiple myeloma patients characterized by the impairment of the plasma cell differentiation have functional B lymphocytes deficiency but T lymphocyte system is not involved. Chronic lymphatic leukemia patients also have significant secondary and often progressive immune deficiencies. In general, more or less severe immunodeficiency is almost always accompanied by malignant neoplasms and lymphoproliferative diseases. Infections are the main cause of mortality in cancer patients, accounting for 50% in patients with solid tumors and lymphomas and in 75% in patients with leukemia.

Secondary immune deficiencies may occur after the administration of immunosuppressive drugs, such as corticosteroids, and some chemotherapeutic agents. The condition of secondary immune deficiency favors the development of recurrent infectious diseases and neoplasms if viral agents are involved in their pathogenesis.

Some immune deficiencies may be associated with other diseases, such as the ataxia-telangiectasia and the Wiskott Aldrich syndrome. The former is characterized by immune deficiency in both the humoral and cell-mediated immunity, ocular and skin telangiectasia, and cerebellar ataxia. The neurologic symptoms consist of deambulation difficulty. At the age of 2–7 years, telangiectatic lesions occur in the bulbar conjunctiva and later extend to the skin. Small patients develop pneumonia and have an increased sensitivity to ionizing radiation, linked to a defect in DNA repair mechanisms.

Wiskott Aldrich syndrome is characterized by recurrent infections, bleeding secondary to thrombocytopenia, and cutaneous eczema that appear during the first months of life. Immune deficiency involves T and B lymphocytes, granulocytes, platelets, and mononuclear phagocytes. This disease is also characterized by the high incidence of associated tumors, in particular non-Hodgkin lymphomas. It is an X-linked recessive inherited congenital immune deficiency and it is therefore transmitted from the mother to the sons. Wiskott Aldrich patients produce antibodies against some microorganisms, such as tetanus, but not against other germs, such as *Hemophilus influenzae or* pneumococci. Due to this defect, infections with these types of bacteria can not normally be defeated; therefore, patients develop frequent recurrent ear infections (otitis), lungs (pneumonia), or even meningitis. T lymphocytes number is normal at birth but progressively decreases over the time. Moreover, T lymphocytes have functional defects. Due to these alterations, patients could develop infections with opportunistic germs such as candida, *Pneumocistis carinii* or herpes virus.

### 4.1.1 AIDS

A particular form of secondary immunodeficiency is AIDS (acquired immunodeficiency syndrome). The syndrome was first reported in literature in 1981, although isolated cases had already been recorded in the 1970s in the United States and in many other areas of the world (Haiti, Africa, and Europe).

In the early 1980, Michael Gottlieb, a researcher at the University of California, was conducting clinical research on immune system deficit and among the patients, he examined a particular case of a young patient suffering of a rare type of pneumonia from *Pneumocistis carinii*, a protozoon that usually affects patients with a weakened immune system. In the following months, Gottlieb discovered three other similar cases, all active homosexuals, with a low level of T lymphocytes. At the end of 1981, the disease still did not have a name. During a congress promoted by FDA in August 1982, it was proposed for the first time the term "acquired immunodeficiency syndrome" for defining this new disease. At the end of 1982 occurred the first death, following an infected transfusion, of a hemophiliac child and the first case of maternal–fetal transmission of AIDS. In May 1983, the virologist Luc Montagnier, at the "Pasteur Institute" of Paris, reported the isolation of a new virus that could be considered the agent responsible for the transmission of the disease. The virus was isolated from cells derived from a homosexual patient with enlarged lymph nodes but without any symptoms of AIDS and cultured in the laboratory. The virus was sent to the Atlanta CDC (Centers for Disease Control and Prevention), analyzed, and named LAV (virus associated with lymphadenopathy), then sent to the National Cancer Institute in Bethesda. On 22 April 1984 the CDC declared that the LAV virus had been definitively identified as the cause of the AIDS by the researchers of the Pasteur Institute. The following day, Margaret Heckler, Secretary of the Health and Human Services, announced that Robert Gallo, director of the National Cancer Institute's Tumor Cell Biology Laboratory, had in turn isolated the virus responsible for the disease from AIDS patients, naming it HTLV -III (human type III T cell leukemia virus).

The HTLVs are the first human retroviruses to be discovered.[3] The declaration also specified that a commercial test would be available to diagnose the infection. A legal battle was engaged between the two prestigious research institutes, which both claimed the paternity of the discovery that was worth the Nobel Prize. In the early months of 1985, different works on the two viruses involved in the dispute were published and later the general conclusion was that the virus were the same. In 1986 an international committee established a new name to indicate the AIDS virus: HIV, or "human immunodeficiency virus."

## 4.2 ANAPHYLAXIS

Anaphylaxis (absence of protection) is a pathophysiological mechanism independent of any inherited factor, while the term of atopy refers to a particular genetic aptitude to produce an excess of IgE directed against different natural substances present in the atmospheric environment, such as pollens and molds, domestic environment, including mites and cockroaches, and even against food.

Anaphylaxis was experimentally demonstrated in 1902 by two French physiologists Paul Portier (1866–1962) and Charles Richet (1850–1935), who showed that the reinoculation of an extract of the tentacles of the sea anemone (*Actinaria*) in dogs already immunized with the same antigen, induced within a few seconds serious disorders that led to their death in a few minutes due to a cardio circulatory collapse syndrome accompanied by bloody diarrhea. The toxin itself was harmless in untreated animals.

In 1905, the American bacteriologist Theobald Smith (1850–1935) observed a similar phenomenon in guinea pigs treated with anti-diphtheria serum mixed with the toxin, to form a nontoxic mixture. The guinea pigs resisted without apparent suffering at the first inoculation but, if the experiment was repeated after some time they died with cardiocirculatory collapse and bronchial asthma. In 1906, the German pathologist Richard Otto showed that the phenomenon did not depend on the toxins activation or a lower resistance acquired towards them, but only by the renewed contact with the antigen.

Later, it was demonstrated that not only the dog and the guinea pigs, but also other animals presented anaphylactic phenomena, which were manifested when the animals were previously treated with a substance with antigenic activity (sensitizing injection) and then inoculated with the same substance (trigger injection).

In 1903, the French immunologist Maurice Arthus (1862–1945) demonstrated that after some subcutaneous injections of horse serum into rabbit, subsequent inoculations resulted in local necrotic lesions. He was studying the production of immune horse antisera in the rabbit by subcutaneous injections and observed that if the horse serum was inoculated for consecutive days, instead of only once, it induced changes that became every day more intense at the injection site. While the first injections were not followed by any local reaction, after 4–5 days it could be observed that the injected liquid was not reabsorbed and caused edema; other injections induced hemorrhagic necrosis and ulceration in the area close to the injection.

In 1905, the Austrian pediatrician Clemens von Pirquet (1874–1924) and his colleague the Hungarian Béla Schick (1877–1967) described serum sickness as a generalized form of the Arthus phenomenon. von Pirquet was trying to combine two apparently contradictory phenomena observed after the exposure to external agents, such as the cow and equine antisera. When he was working with Schick at the Paediatric Department in Vienna, in the wards of children hospitalized with scarlet fever, he noted that some patients who had received the antiserum, developed a spectrum of systemic and local symptoms, especially fever, rash, arthropathy, and swollen lymph nodes, which Schick and von Pirquet named "serum sickness." Similar symptoms observed after diphtheria and tetanus antiserum administration appeared in the previously admitted patient medical records. Therefore the serum therapy seemed to have produced not only immunity (protection) but also hypersensitivity (or "supersensitivity," as they preferred to call it). Von Pirquet realized that in both situations the serum, an external agent, induced in the organism some form of "modified or altered reactivity" for which he proposed the term *allergy*.

During sero-therapeutic treatments in humans, the first serotherapy induced the production of antibodies against horse (that was the most used animal for the preparation of curative sera) serum proteins and if the same person after some time received a second serotherapy he was subjected to extremely serious anaphylactic shock that could lead to the death if the necessary preventive measures were not implemented (use of the serum of another animal or dealbuminized serum).

## 4.3 IMMEDIATE HYPERSENSITIVITY

In 1926, the American bacteriologist Arthur F. Coca (1875–1959), founder of the Journal of Immunology, suggested to not use the term *allergy* on the basis of its different and conflicting meanings. He did not consider "anaphylaxis" as a part of the allergy because it was a phenomenon in which the antigen–antibody reaction was fixed. Instead, he categorized as allergy all those conditions in which he believed that an antibody mechanism had not been demonstrated, for example in drug "idiosyncrasies," in serum sickness in humans, and in hay fever. In fact, the concept of "allergy" referring to all hypersensitivity forms except for anaphylaxis would remain until the 1940s.

In the 1960s, the British immunologist Robin Coombs (1921–2006) and the English pathologist Philip Gell (1914–2001) tried to restore the original meaning to the term *allergy*. They noticed that "hypersensitivity" is a general term used for describing an adverse clinical reaction against an antigen (or allergen). The antigen could be bacterial-derived, such as in a classical reaction of delayed type hypersensitivity to the tuberculin, or allergen-derived, as an IgE-mediated hypersensitivity to pollen. They supposed that limiting the term *allergy* to describe any exaggerated response of the immune system to external substances was illogical since the role of the immune system is to produce immunity, by definition. A large part of this difficulty is removed if instead of "allergy" we refer to "allergic diseases" and we confine the word allergy (as von Pirquet originally intended) to a nonspecific biological response. In the individual this nonspecific response can lead to both immunity (which produces benefits) or allergic disease (which is harmful).

In 1966, the Japanese Kimishige Ishizaka (1925–) isolated from the sera derived by a pool of allergopathic patients a molecular fraction containing the reaginic antibodies, then proceeded with an enrichment and the immunization of experimental animals. In this way an antiserum absolutely specific towards the reaginic antibodies was obtained. Ishizaka established the immunoglobulin nature of these antibodies belonging to a class different from those known up until then, called IgE.

In 1969, a case of myeloma was described in which the monoclonal myelomatous protein presented atypical properties with respect to the known immunoglobulin classes, and it was named ND from the patient's initials. Subsequently, it was possible to establish the perfect identity between the two molecules (Bennich et al., 1989).

Michael A. Kaliner and Rober P. Orange at the National Institute of Allergy and Infectious Diseases, together with K. Frank Austen from Harvard Medical School, and Teruko Ishizaka from John Hopkins University, in the 1970s, clarified the events sequence leading to mast cells degranulation. IgE are secreted by a plasma cell in response to the first appearance of an antigen and then fixed to the mast cells plasma membrane receptors. When a new antigen exposure occurs, the antigen epitopes bind to two adjacent IgE molecules. The formation of a bridge between the IgE molecules triggers the degranulation of the mast cells and the release of the intracellular chemical mediators.

These chemical mediators are able to induce the bronchial smooth muscle cells contraction, to dilate the wall of the small blood vessels and to increase its permeability, to stimulate the secretion of the mucous glands, and to activate the platelets. Once the chemical mediators are released, they can be neutralized by drugs such as antihistamines and aspirin, or their activity can be countered by products such as adrenaline.

In addition to the preformed chemical mediators, contained in the mast cells granules are newly-formed mediators, the prostaglandins and the leukotrienes, both deriving from the arachidonic acid. The structure of leukotrienes was determined in the 1970s by Bengt Samuelsson at the Karolinska Institute in Stockholm, who was awarded the Nobel Prize for Medicine in 1982 for this discovery.

## 4.4 DELAYED HYPERSENITIVITY

In 18th-century Europe, smallpox poisoning was practiced. This consisted of inducing smallpox in an attenuated form by the scarification with pustules removed from the sick. Voltaire, who survived a smallpox attack at the age of 29, was a convinced supporter of the inoculation, but another supporter was especially a mathematician and geographer, Charles Marie de la Condamine, who considered the poisoning as a useful means for controlling outbreak.

In 1798, the English physician Edward Jenner finalized the first vaccine. In England in his time it was usual to use the smallpox inoculation, a procedure by which the small wound to be immunized, specially created in the subject, was sprinkled with the material coming from pustules of sick individuals. By doing so, the subject developed a mild smallpox that made him immune to the real illness. This practice, however, was dangerous to the health of patients, family, and acquaintances until his recovery.

Jenner noticed that in previously vaccinated subjects, an erythematous skin reaction developed at the site of a new vaccine virus inoculation, reaching its maximum intensity within 24–72 hours. Jenner worked in a region where cattle breeding was widespread and noted that during a smallpox outbreak there was an important proportion of resistant individuals among cattle farmers. Instead, they were subject to contracting vaccine smallpox, very common among cattle. He demonstrated how the inoculation of bovine smallpox (or bovine vaccine) in humans was able to confer protection against human smallpox. Jenner sent an article to the Royal Society of London, in which he described 13 cases of subjects immunized with bovine smallpox, but the Royal Society refused to publish it. Jenner later published it at his own expense. The method was dubbed "vaccination" by Jenner because the original serum was of vaccine origin and the results of its experience were published in 1798 under the title *An Inquiry into the Causes and Effects of the Variolae Vaccinae, a Disease Known by the Name of Cow Pox.*[4]

Throughout the 1800s the only available vaccine was that against smallpox. Only at the end of the century did Louis Pasteur guess that this practice (vaccination) to be effective and harmless required the inoculation of attenuated pathogens and that it could be extended to other infectious diseases: in 1881 he vaccinated the sheep against the carbuncle and in 1885 administered the first rabies vaccine to an Alsatian boy who had been repeatedly bitten by a dog suffering from the disease.

In 1890, Robert Koch[5] demonstrated that with the injection of live tuberculous bacilli in already infected guinea pigs skin after 24 hours a dark nodule appeared and subsequently it turned into a necrotic ulcer ("Koch phenomenon"). In uninfected animals the injected area was not detectable and was healed with a small nodule. Koch is responsible for the formulation of the so-called "Koch postulates" according to which: (a) the bacterium must be present in all cases of the disease; (b) the bacterium must be isolated in culture and maintained in subsequent subcultures; (c) the same bacterium, kept in culture, if injected into receptive animals must determine a characteristic pathology associated to constant and reproducible anatomical pathological findings; and (d) the same bacterium must be present and then isolated again from the experimentally infected animal. Over time a gradual reevaluation of Koch's statements has occurred, in particular the criteria to be considered in the recognition of the etiological determinant role of a microorganism as an agent of a disease must comply with Koch's dictates, supplemented by other checks that take into account direct diagnostic procedures (detection of toxins and virulence factors, molecular tests) and indirect (humoral and cellular immune responses).

The first clinical use of the Koch phenomenon was reported in 1891 by the observation that the skin reaction to tuberculin could be reproduced into the child and this test could be used in the infantile tuberculosis diagnosis (Epstein, 1891). In 1908, The French researcher Charles E. M. Mantoux (1877–1947) introduced the method of intradermal injection of the tuberculin (Mantoux reaction), widely adopted later in clinical diagnostics. In 1925, the US bacteriologist Hans Zinsser (1878–1940) specified that the reaction to tuberculin could occur without any demonstrable circulating antibodies and he named this reaction "delayed hypersensitivity" or "bacterial allergy" because it appeared during other bacterial diseases.

In 1942, Landsteiner and the immunologist Merril W. Chase (1905–2004) passively transferred a skin reaction from delayed hypersensitivity to picryl chloride in guinea pigs by using leukocytes obtained from the peritoneal exudate of sensitized leukocytes. In 1945, Chase extended this observation to the tuberculin skin reaction, transferring skin sensitivity with the use of peritoneal exudate leucocytes of tuberculin-positive guinea pigs. Later, it was possible to demonstrate the same effect using peripheral blood and lymph node leukocytes.

## 4.5 AUTOIMMUNITY

At the beginning of the 20th century, despite the existence of sporadic experimental researches such as those on antisperm antibodies, and those regarding the hemolytic anemia, the paroxysmal cold hemoglobinuria,[6] knowledge on autoimmunity was very limited. In 1956, it was discovered in the serum of patients with Hashimoto's[7] thyroiditis the presence of antibodies capable of reacting with thyroglobulin (Roitt et al., 1956).

Since Roitt and colleagues noticed the decline in serum gamma globulin following the thyroid removal in Hashimoto's thyroiditis, they verified the hypothesis that the plasma cells present in the gland produced an autoantibody against a thyroid component, thus causing tissue damage and chronic inflammatory response. The serum of the first analyzed patients presented antibodies directed against normal thyroid extracts autoantigen, identified in thyroglobulin.

In 1956, the possibility was also demonstrated to reproduce thyroid lesions in experimental animals similar to human thyroiditis, through the immunization obtained with homologous thyroglobulin emulsified in Freund's complete adjuvant (Rose and Witebsky, 1956). The adjuvant triggers a chronic inflammation at the injection site leading to the destruction of the gland follicular structure which accumulate lymphocytes and cells presenting the antigen to specific lymphocytes which, in turn, are activated to induce a thyroiditis at a distance. In 1957, it was recognized in the serum of patients with Basedow's disease[8] the presence of factors stimulating the thyroid functional activity, subsequently identified as autoantibodies directed towards epitopes associated with the thyroid receptor for TSH (Adams and Purves, 1957).

In 1962, the criteria for autoimmune diseases were defined (Milgrom and Witebski, 1962), subsequently reviewed, and integrated in 1993 (Rose and Bona, 1993). An unhealthy condition can be defined as autoimmune when it meets these criteria: demonstration of humoral and/or cell-mediated autoimmune responses; recognition of a specific antigen against which autoimmune responses are addressed; induction of an autoimmune response against the same antigen and reproduction in the experimental animal the lesions found in the human pathology; passive transport of the disease by serum containing autoantibodies or by self-reactive immunocompetent cells. The application of these criteria made it possible to establish that more than 80 diseases previously with unknown etiology could be included in this group and that all the organs or systems could be affected.

Autoimmune diseases are currently classified into organ-specific autoimmune diseases and systemic autoimmune diseases; in the former (such as type I diabetes mellitus, autoimmune hemolytic anemia, and myasthenia gravis) the aggression target to the immune system is contained in a single organ; in the latter (such as rheumatoid arthritis, systemic lupus erythematosus and scleroderma), more organs and tissues are affected by the disease.

The progress of knowledge in the field of autoimmunity derived from the use and improvement of methods for the detection of humoral and/or cellular responses towards autoantigens (immunofluorescence, immunoperoxidase assay, radioimmunoassay methods, inhibition of leukocyte migration, in vitro blast transformation), and animal models.

While Burnet developed the clonal selection theory, he hypothesized either the autoantigen was excluded by the immune system or the potential antibody-forming cells, when prematurely exposed to autoantigen during their ontogenetic development, were removed or inactivated. In this context the autoimmunity was considered due to the proliferation of the so-called "prohibited clones" of lymphocytes with a specificity to the autoantigen.

In opposition to the excluded antigens hypothesis, Torrigiani and collaborators, in 1969, showed that thyroglobulin was present in human serum in normal conditions at concentrations ranging from 10 to 100 ng/mL. In 1986, Avrameas demonstrated the presence, in normal human, rat, and mouse serum, of autoantibodies called natural autoantibodies capable of reacting with a wide variety of autoantigens, such as thyroglobulin, actin, myosin, myoglobin, spectrin, and myelin basic protein. In 1968, Mitchison demonstrated that low doses of an antigen induced in a mouse injected with bovine serum albumin or with gamma globulin, the lack of response (tolerance) of T helper lymphocytes, leaving intact the response ability of B lymphocytes. At high doses, however, it induces a lack of response in both B and T lymphocytes (the phenomenon of low and high area tolerance).

There are several immunopathogenetic mechanisms through which autoimmune responses can occur: type II immunoreactions (cytolytic or cytotoxic), due to antibodies able to react with surface antigens, such as those expressed by blood cells; of type III, by formation and deposition of antigen–antibody complexes able to activate the complement; or of type IV (from delayed or cell-mediated hypersensitivity) by activation of cytotoxic T lymphocytes.[9]

Genetic, immunological, and environmental components are the conditions promoting autoimmunity. It is known that the susceptibility to autoimmune diseases is influenced by some genes of the HLA complex, whose products or molecules of class I and II are able to selectively bind autoantigens and present them to autoreactive T cells which, through an altered cytokines secretion, induce the autoimmune disease. Some diseases correlate with class I genes (ankylosing spondylitis, Behcet's syndrome, reactive arthritis), most of them correlate with class II genes (DR, DP, DQ). Sometimes only one gene, or at other times more HLA genes confer susceptibility to autoimmune diseases, for example, type I diabetes mellitus, Hashimoto's thyroiditis, systemic lupus erythematosus (LES), scleroderma, hepatitis, rheumatoid arthritis, celiac disease. Among the environmental factors, iodine, a critical element for the synthesis of thyroid hormones, is an environmental risk factor for the onset of autoimmune diseases affecting the thyroid.

In this context, in the 1980s, the immunologist Gianfranco Bottazzo, working at Middlesex Hospital in London, showed that normal cultured thyroid cells expressed class II molecules after stimulation with mitogens. Applying the direct immunofluorescence technique by anti-DR monoclonal antibodies it was then possible to demonstrate the presence of class II molecules in thyroid follicular cells of patients with Hashimoto's thyroiditis or with Basedow's disease. The presence of class II molecules was confirmed in $\beta$-insular cells in type I diabetes mellitus, in salivary duct cells in Sjögren's syndrome, and in bile duct cells in primary biliary cirrhosis. Bottazzo envisaged a general theory of autoimmunity according to which the ectopic expression of class II molecules on the epithelial cells would make them able to present their own membrane autoantigens to self-reactive helper T cells.

Autoimmune diseases can in part be prevented by vaccination with viral antigens that do not trigger autoimmune reactions. R.M. Zinkernagel, at the Institute of Experimental Immunology at the University of Zurich, vaccinated transgenic mice with a lymphocyte meningitis virus antigen and then he infected the mice with the virus. He demonstrated that T lymphocytes activated against the vaccine antigen are able to eliminate the virus before the occurrence of the autoimmune reaction and before the mice become diabetic (the mice become diabetic when they are infected by the virus without having been vaccinated).

The first efforts of immunotherapy in some of the most important autoimmune diseases, such as systemic lupus erythematosus, rheumatoid arthritis, and progressive systemic sclerosis, date back to the 1960s. These groundbreaking immunotherapy approaches were based on widely empiric criteria such as the use of levamisole, an anthelmintic drug able to modulate in vitro the activity of T and B lymphocytes, and the *transfer factor*, a lymphocytic extract potential nonspecific immunity inducer, used in some lymphomas and in Wiskott Aldrich syndrome. Immunosuppression represents the most valid therapeutic approach in the treatment of autoimmune diseases until today.

The spreading of autoimmune diseases is significantly increasing in the world population. The causes of this increase are not known, but the most suggestive hypothesis supposes that the increase of autoimmune outbreaks is the result of the decreased activity of the immune system against the nonself as a consequence of the reduced incidence of infectious diseases in the population.

## ENDNOTES

1. In 1832, the pathologist Thomas Hodgkin, describing seven patients who died with splenomegaly and systemic lymphadenopathy, first focused his attention on a disease of the lymphoreticular system that he named Hodgkin's disease. In 1898, the pathologist Carl Sternberg, illustrating the clinical and histopathological case histories of 15 patients, underlined the concept according to which the diagnosis of this disease had to be based essentially on histological investigation. In 1902, the pathologist Dorothy Reed described the characteristic giant cells with one or more nuclei, later referred to as Reed–Stenberg cells.

2. Tumors of the lymphatic system could be considered as the consequence of abnormalities of thymus development. In 1956, Jacob Furth, of the Oak Ridge National Laboratory, was the first to demonstrate that the early thymus removal prevented the development of a lymphoma that appears spontaneously in certain strains of mice. On the other hand, Peterson and Ben R. Burmester, at the East Lansing Department of Agriculture in Michigan, demonstrated in 1964 that bursectomy, and not thymectomy, prevented the development of virus-induced lymphoma in chickens.

3. The peculiarity of retroviruses is to reverse the normal genetic information flow, ranging from DNA to RNA and proteins. The retrovirus genetic material is constituted by RNA, and the retrovirus carries an enzyme called reverse transcriptase that uses viral RNA as a template for DNA production. In this way the viral DNA can be integrated into the host's genome.

4. The intensive program for of smallpox eradication was launched by WHO on January 1, 1967 and the success of the global campaign based on surveillance and containment of the virus resulted that, in the 1970s, smallpox was confined to the Horn of Africa alone, with the last report of a case, in Somalia, in 1977. The world announcement by WHO of the eradication of smallpox at the planetary level dates back to 1980.

5. Robert Koch (1843–1910) was a German physician, bacteriologist, and microbiologist. He was the first to describe the role of a pathogen in the genesis of a disease by discovering the pathogenic agent of tuberculosis (*Mycobacterium tuberculosis*). His contributions to the study of infectious diseases were numerous.

6. In this pathological condition that depends on the production of hemolysins directed against its own red blood cells an intravascular hemolysis accompanied by urinary elimination of hemoglobin occurs.

7. The first description of autoimmune chronic thyroiditis dates back to 1912, when Hakaru Hashimoto reported the cases of four women, all aged over 40 years and of whom at least one clinically hypothyroid, who had undergone thyroidectomy for goiter. Hashimoto's thyroiditis occurs with a volumetric increase in the thyroid (goiter), hypothyroidism, or both. The reduced function of the gland depends on a progressive atrophy of the thyroid follicles, which are widely infiltrated by B and T lymphocytes, and by plasma cells. In addition, Hashimoto's thyroiditis promotes the development of B-cell lymphomas.

8. Graves–Basedow disease is caused by the presence of autoantibodies stimulating and activating the TSH receptor which in turn causes the increase in the synthesis and secretion of thyroid hormones and therefore cause the onset of diffuse goiter. It has been demonstrated in vitro that the lymphocytes present in the thyroid tissue spontaneously produce autoantibodies.

9. The first classification of hypersensitivity reactions, based on the effector immune mechanism as cause of the disease, was formulated in 1963 and it included four types of reaction. Type I

includes the usual anaphylactic and allergic or atopic reactions; the type II includes the cyto-toxic and cytolytic reactions caused by the activation of the complement system and phagocy-tosis, following the interaction between the antibody and cellular antigens; the type III includes the pathogenic reactions mediated by immune complexes that, in mild excess of antigen, precipitate in the tissues activating the complement and releasing chemotactic and permeabilizing mediators; the type IV includes immunological reactions mediated by T lym-phocytes specifically sensitized. Unlike the first three reactions, which can be passively trans-ferred with the serum, the latter can be transferred only by inoculation of the T lymphocytes of a donor previously sensitized. In the determinism of these reactions, the release of cytokines is fundamental and the lesions are characterized by a lymphocytic or lympho-macrophage infiltrate, which is responsible for the tissue damage. The classification of Gell and Coombs was extended in 1971, with the description of the V-type reactions (stimulatory hypersensitiv-ity) induced by antireceptor antibodies, which have an agonist action that mimics the effector action of the physiological ligand. Subsequently the reactions of type VI from Irvine and of VII type were also described. The reactions of type VI concerns antibodies and killer cells-mediated cytotoxic reactions, while the reactions of VII type, which take place in myasthenia gravis and in pernicious anemia, are induced by the action of inhibitory antibodies which, interacting with the hormone and neurotransmitters cellular receptors, inhibit the action of the physiological ligand causing a serious deficit of the functional activity.

# CHAPTER 5

# Immunity and Tumors: The Surveillance Theory

Tumor immunology has always been intimately correlated to the transplantation immunology. The possibility to utilize genetically homogeneous strains of animals has allowed the establishment of the immunogenetic principles of transplantation biology. Tumor cells have both histocompatibility antigens and tumor transplant antigens, both strongly immunogenic. Therefore, specific tumor immunity can only be studied in strains of genetically homogeneous, singular, or identical twins.

The frequency of tumors in subjects suffering from a primary immunological deficience is higher than that of the normal population. Tumors that occur in subjects with late immunological deficiencies, which affect cellular and humoral immunity, consist of gastric and colon carcinomas, epitheliomas, reticulum sarcomas, lymphomas, and leukemia. Aging is also associated with the weakening of immunological functions and the increase in the frequency of tumors.

The concept of immunity surveillance against tumors was first formulated in 1941 by the American Geneticist Clearance C. Little (1888–1971), who claimed that transplant rejection is the basis of the immune response and suggested that the immune system plays an important role in carcinogenesis. In 1954 it was demonstrated that a carcinogen, through the formation of a complex with an antigen on the cell surface, became itself immunogenic and the consequent immune reaction inactivated it depriving cells of the malignancy characteristics (Green, 1954). In 1957, it was demonstrated that inbred (genetically identical) mice could be immunized against carcinogen-induced tumors, thus proving the existence of tumor-specific antigens (Prehn and Main, 1957).

In 1970, Frank Mac Farlane Burnet developed the suggestions that the American pathologist Lewis Thomas expressed in 1959 in a speech at a fringe event of a conference that Peter Medawar had held in the context of a congress on the general aspects of delayed

Immunology in the Twentieth Century. DOI: https://doi.org/10.1016/B978-0-12-816145-6.00005-6

hypersensitivity. Thomas believed that the biological mechanisms involved in transplant rejection could also be the basis of natural defenses against the onset of tumors. Burnet elaborated the theory of immune surveillance, whose assumptions are fundamentally two: neo-plastic cells derive from normal cells by mutation, express different membrane antigens (neo-antigens) with respect to normal cells and are recognized as foreign by the immune system that processes a cell-mediated response with the aim of eliminating them, similarly to what happens in the transplant rejection. The onset of a tumor would be due to inadequate immune surveillance, such as that occurring in elderly subjects and in immunodeficiency conditions. At the base of the theory of immune surveillance there is the consideration on the adaptive meaning in immune responses.

After the wording of the theory, several tumor-specific antigens were identified and characterized.

Phren performed a historic experiment demonstrating that if in a mouse affected by methylcolanthene-induced sarcoma the tumor was removed and then reimplanted in the same animal, the tumor did not grow but was rejected, while it grew if implanted in a syngeneic animal. The hypothesis was formulated that the tumor-affected mouse was sensitized by the presence of antigens expressed by the tumor and developed an immune response that was responsible for rejection following the second implant (Phren and Main, 1957).

Every tumor possesses an individual antigen that corresponds to a mutant endogen protein. The most powerful carcinogens, in particular those that induce a fast neoplastic transformation, tend to evoke power tumor antigens. Some tumors produce fetal and embryonic antigens, such as alpha-fetus protein or the carcinoembryonic antigen. The first human tumor antigen (MAGE-1) was identified and isolated from a melanoma in 1991 (Van der Bruggen et al., 1991).

In the decade following the formulation of the immune surveillance theory against tumors, numerous studies were conducted to enhance the possible immunological antitumor defenses. The immune system was stimulated with autologous or allergenic tumor cell extracts or with nonspecific preparations such as bacillus Calmette-Guerin (BCG)[1] and *Corynebacterium parvum* (CP) or with chemicals such as dinitrochlorobenzene.

Numerous subsequent clinical and experimental evidences challenged the theory of immune surveillance. It has been shown that carcinogenesis is a multiphase process and that oncogenes play a decisive role in this process. The neoplastic cell population is extremely heterogeneous and the phenotypic heterogeneity is reflected in an extreme variability of the antigenic characteristics of the various subpopulations of neoplastic cells. It follows that it becomes extremely difficult to predict a specific immune response to a specific neoplasm. Furthermore, the increase in the incidence of tumors in immunocompromised individuals is related to tumors such as lymphomas, Kaposi's sarcoma, and cutaneous carcinomas. Otherwise, the incidence of the most common tumors, such as breast, lung, and intestinal carcinomas is not changed in immunocompromised individuals. It has been shown that nude mice lacking functioning thymus and effective cell-mediated responses do not have an increased susceptibility to chemical carcinogenesis processes (Stutman, 1975).

The tumor immune response is not mediated only from T lymphocytes as the immune surveillance theory supports, but also B lymphocytes, macrophages, and NK cells contribute through a combined and coordinated action. The tumoricidal activity of NK cells is increased by cytokines, such a IL-2 and IL-12 and interferons. In the past, IL-2 has been used to activate the NK cells derived from the neoplastic patients, generating the lymphokine activated killer cells, which were then reinfused. Macrophages also have the ability to kill cancer cells, both through their Fc receptors that bind tumor surface antibodies (mechanism of cytotoxicity dependent antibody, ADCC), and through lytic mediators, such as nitric oxide and tumor necrosis factor.

There are different mechanisms through which tumors can bypass the immune response ("immunoevasion"). The tumor may have lost the expression of tumor antigens or may have a reduced expression of MHC class I molecules. Furthermore, patients with advanced tumors have a reduced NK cell-mediated cytotoxic activity and a decreased production of nitric oxide by macrophages.

Immuno-oncology is based on the awareness that a targeted and effective immune response against a specific type of cancer can lead to significant clinical benefits in patients. Immuno-oncology has started a new era in tumors treatment, so it is important to deepen the action mechanisms of this new type of treatment, which complement the "classic" weapons available until now (surgery, chemotherapy, radio-therapy, target therapies). Compared to treatment with target thera-pies, an immuno-oncological drug does not generate visible results immediately, since it does not directly affect the tumor cells, but acti-vates the immune system to obtain the desired response.

Another important difference with respect to "classic" therapies is that, over time, they can select tumor cell strains with greater drug resistance, resulting in a rapid evolution of the neoplasm. In the case of immunotherapy, however, thus it does not act directly on the tumor cell, but on the immune system, this selection does not occur and, even in case of disease progression, the evolution tends to be slower.

Melanoma has become the ideal experimental model for the devel-opment of new immuno-oncology drugs. In order to treat this highly aggressive and resistant to the usual treatment tumor, a new class of therapeutic agents has been developed such as the so-called immuno-modulating monoclonal antibodies. The progenitor of these drugs is ipilimumab, which acts on the CTLA-4 receptor (antigen 4 associated with cytotoxic T lymphocytes). The CTLA-4 plays an important role in the protection against autoimmune diseases and immunosuppression during tumorigenesis. When CTLA-4 binds to the molecule B7 the inhibitory signal activated interrupts the immune system activation. As a consequence, blocking the molecule through a monoclonal anti-CTLA-4 antibody prevents the B7-CTLA-4 binding which, by remov-ing the inhibitory signal, reactivates and enhances the immune response. Ipilimumab was initially approved in Europe in July 2011 by the European Medicines Agency, for use in patients with metastatic melanoma who had received prior therapy.

## ENDNOTE

1. The BCG is generally administered by intradermic multiple inoculations or subcutaneously or directly into the tumor mass. In some therapeutic protocols, BCG was inoculated in associa-tion with tumor cells previously surgically excised.

# CHAPTER 6

# Conclusions

During the 20th century our knowledge in the immunological field had an impressive acceleration. Until the 1930s, immune phenomena were considered as the expression of a single interaction type, between antibody and antigen. The observation and study of the phenomena associated with the acquisition of immunity from infections led to the development of new technical and cognitive tools that favored further development of knowledge in this area.

A series of basic immunology knowledge going back to the 1950s appears to be of great biological significance. We are reminded only of a few: those on antibodies, on lymphocytes, on macrophages, on the complement; the expansion of lymphocyte clones in response to antigen; the immunological memory; the subdivision of lymphocytes into B lymphocytes and T lymphocytes. From the 1960s to the present day, the number of immunologists enrolled in the golden register of researchers who have been awarded the Nobel Prize for Medicine or Physiology has increased at close intervals.

Basic immunology developed close relationships with the most diverse sectors of basic biological sciences such as chemistry, biochemistry, pathological anatomy, genetics, microbiology, molecular biology, and pharmacology. Thanks to interdisciplinary researches, it has been possible to achieve some important advancements, such as concerning the immunoglobulins structure, immunogenetics, the different lymphocyte subpopulations characterization, the molecular bases of immune response. The immune system has proven to be not only a defense system, but also a recognition system, which allows it to differentiate what is the self from what is non-self.

The ability to recognize the antigen and to keep memory of the meeting depends on a selection process of cells induced to differentiate and synthesize a specific antibody. There is an unlimited repertoire of antibodies to deal with the wide range of antigens present in the environment (the epitope universe). Thus a "Darwinian" hypothesis joined

Immunology in the Twentieth Century. DOI: https://doi.org/10.1016/B978-0-12-816145-6.00006-8

"immunology," regarding the selection similar to the species adaptive changes to the environment.

In this book we have tried to provide a measure of the central role played by the immunological research in the field of biomedical sciences and how its advancements involve seemingly distant disciplines, such as mathematics, philosophy, and psychology. Frank Macfarlane Burnet, one of the most important immunologists of the 20th century, believed that immunology was a more philosophical than practical science.

At the same time, immunology has become a crucial medical discipline. The greatest success of immunology in medicine has been the practice of vaccination. All organs can be targets of immune aggression. Vertebrates have developed more defense mechanisms compared to those of the innate immunity, which correspond to the so-called adaptive immunity, a process that is constantly evolving during the life of an individual.

The progress of immunological knowledge has given rise to clinical immunology and allergology. Transplant rejection depends fundamentally on immunological phenomena. Immune system involvement in tumor growth is one of the most important models to study in oncology; moreover, immunotherapy, now back in vogue, has joined the more traditional chemotherapy and radiation therapy in the tumors treatment. The deepening knowledge at the molecular and gene level has allowed the realization of more rational and effective therapeutic strategies.

In this new millennium the perspective is to bring further new knowledge within this discipline, the immunology, at the same time so fascinating and complex, that allows us to face in a more rational and effective manner the treatment of human diseases, from the simplest ones to those still today, unfortunately, incurable.

# REFERENCES

Adams, D.D., Purves, H.D., 1957. The role of tyrotrophin in hypertyroidism and exophtalmos. Metabolism 6, 26–35.

Alexander, J., 1932. Some intracellular aspects of life and diseases. Protoplasma 14, 296–306.

Barnes, D.W., Loutit, J.F., 1957. Treatment of murine leukaemia with x-rays and homologous bone marrow. Bri. J. Haematol. 3, 241–252.

Bennich, H., Ishizaka, K., Ishizaka, T., Johansson, S.G., 1989. A comparative antigenic study of gamma-e globulin and myeloma-IgND. J. Immunol. 102, 826–831.

Bordet, J., 1899. Agglutination et dissolution des globules rouges par le serum: deuxieme mémoire. Ann. l'Institut Pasteur 13, 273–297.

Breinl, F., Haurowitz, F.Z., 1930. Chemische Untersuchung des Präzipitates aus Hämoglobin und Anti-Hämoglobinserum und Bemerkungen über die Natur des Antikörper. Zeitschrift für physiologische Chemie 192, 45.

Bruton, O., 1952. Agammaglobulinemia. Pediatrics 9, 722–728.

Burnet, F.M., 1957. A modification of Jerne's theory of antibody production using the concept of clonal selection. Aust. J. Sci. 20, 67–68.

Burnet, F.M., 1959. The Clonal Selection Theory of Acquired Immunity. Cambridge University Press, Cambridge.

Burnet, F.M., 1967. Le difese organiche. Boringhieri, Torino.

Burnet, F.M., Fenner, F., 1941. The Production of Antibodies, second ed MacMillan, Melbourne, p. 1949.

Burnet, F.M., Fenner, F., 1948. Genetics and immunology. Heredity 2, 289–324.

Celada, F. (Ed.), 1992. La nuova immunologia. Le Scienze Editore, Milano.

Chase, M.W., 1945. Cellular transfer of cutaneous hypersensitivity to tuberculin. Proc. Soc. Exp. Biol. Med. 59, 134–135.

Cleveland, W.W., Fogel, B.J., Brown, W.T., Kay, H.E., et al., 1968. Foetal thymic transplants in a case of Di George's syndrome. Lancet 2, 1211–1214.

Corbellini, G., 1990. L'evoluzione del pensiero immunologico. Bollati Boringhieri, Torino.

Corbellini, G., 1996. In: Bellone, E., Mangione, C. (Eds.), Il sistema immunitario, L. Geymonat, Storia del pensiero filosofico e scientifico, vol. IX. Garzanti, Milano, pp. 254–285.

Di George, A., 1968. Congenital absence of the thymus and its immunological consequences: concurrence with congenital hypoparathyroidism. In: Bergsma, D., Good, R.A. (Eds.), Immunologic Deficiency Diseases in Man. Williams and Wilkins, Baltimore.

Dreyer, W.J., Bennett, J.C., 1965. The molecular basis of antibody formation: a paradox. Proc. Nat. Acad. Sci. USA 54, 864–869.

Edelman, G.M., 1959. Dissociation of $\gamma$-globulin. J. Am. Chem. Soc. 81, 3155.

Edmonds, R.H., 1966. Electron microscopy of erythropoiesis in the avian yolk sac. Anat. Rec. 154, 785–805.

Ehrlich, P., 1900. On immunity with special reference to cell life. Proc. Royal Soc. (Series B) 66, 424–448.

Ehrlich, W.E., Harris, T.N., 1942. The formation of antibodies in the popliteal lymph nodes in rabbits. J. Exp. Med. 76, 335–347.

Epstein, A., 1891. Ueber die Anwendung Koch'scher injectionen in Säuglingsund ersten kindesalter. Prog. Medizinische Wochenschrift 16, 13.

Ford, C.E., Micklem, H.S., 1974. The thymus and lymph nodes in radiation chimeras. Lancet 16, 359–362.

Gershon, R.K., Kondo, K., 1970. Cell interactions in the induction of tolerance: the role of thymic lymphocytes. Immunology 18, 723–737.

Gershon, R.K., Gery, I., Waksman, B.H., 1974. Suppressive effects of in vivo immunization on pha responses in vitro. J. Immunol. 112, 215–221.

Gitlin, D., Janeway, C.A., 1956. Agammaglobulinemia: congenital, acquired and transient forms. Prog. Hematol. 1, 318–329.

Glanzmann, E., Riniker, P., 1950. Essential lymphocytopoiesis, new clinical aspects of infant pathology. Ann. Ped. 175, 1–32.

Good, R.A., Zack, S.J., 1956. Disturbances in gamma globulin synthesis as experiments of nature. Pediatrics 18, 109–149.

Good, R.A., Mac Lean, L.D., Varco, R.L., Zak, S.J., 1956. Thymic tumor and acquired agammaglobulinemia: a clinical and experimental study of the immune response. Surgery 40, 1010–1017.

Good, R.A., Kelly, W.D., Rotstein, J., Varco, R.L., et al., 1962. Immunological deficiency diseases. Agammaglobulinemia, hypogammaglobulinemia, Hodgkin's disease and sarcoidosis. Prog. Allergy 6, 187–319.

Gordon, J., Mac Lean, L.D., 1965. A lymphocyte-stimulating factor produced in vitro. Nature 208, 795–796.

Green, E.U., 1954. Effects of hydrocarbon-protein conjugates on frog embryos. I. Arrest of development by conjugates of 9,10-dimethyl-1,2-benzanthracene. Cancer Res. 14, 591–598.

Green, H.N., 1954. An immunological concept of cancer: a preliminary report. Bri. Med. J. 2, 1374–1380.

Haskins, K., Kubo, R., White, J., Pigeon, M., Kappler, J., Marrack, P., et al., 1983. The major histocompatibility complex-restricted antigen receptor T cells. Isolation with a monoclonal antibody. J. Exp. Med. 157, 1149–1169.

Hellman, T., 1930. Lymphgefässe, lymphknötchen, und lymphnoten. In: Von Möllendorff, W. (Ed.), In Handbuch der microskopischen anatomie des menschen. Springer, Berlin, pp. 328–346.

Kasakura, S., Lowenstein, L., 1965. A factor stimulating DNA synthesis derived from the medium of leukocyte cultures. Nature 208, 794–795.

Koch, R., 1890. Weitere Mitteilungen über ein Heilmittel gegen Tuberkulose. Deutsche Medizinische Wochenschrift 16, 29.

Levine, P., Stetson, R.E., 1939. An unusual case of intragroup agglutination. J. Am. Med. Assoc. 113, 126.

Little, C.C., 1941. The genetics of tumor transplantation. In: Snell, G.D. (Ed.), Biology of the Laboratory Mouse. Blakiston, Philadelphia.

Maximov, A.A., 1924. Relation of blood cells to connective tissues and endothelium. Physiol. Rev. 4, 533–563.

Mc Master, P.D., Hudack, S.S., 1935. The formation of agglutinins within lymph nodes. J. Exp. Med. 61, 783–792.

Medawar, P.B., 1944. The behavior and fate of skin autografts and skin homografts in rabbits. J. Anat. 78, 176–199.

Medawar, P.B., 1945. A second study of the behavior and fate of kin homografts in rabbits: a report of the War wounds committee of the Medical Research Council. J. Anat. 79, 157–176.

Medawar, P.B., 1958. The homograft reaction. Proc. Royal Soc. London B 149, 145.

Milgrom, F., Witebski, E., 1962. Autoantibodies and autoimmune diseases. J. Am. Med. Association 181, 706–716.

Miller, J.F.A.P., 1961. Immunological function of the thymus. Lancet 2, 748–749.

Miller, J.F.A.P., Basten, A., Sprent, J., Cheers, C., 1971. Interation between lymphocytes in immune response. Cell. Immunol. 2, 469–495.

Mitchison, N.A., 1968. The dosage requirements for immunological paralysis by soluble proteins. Immunology 15, 509–530.

Mitchison, N.A., 1970. Mechanisms of action of anti-lymphocyte serum. FASEB J. 29, 222–223.

Mitechell, G.F., Miller, J.F.A.P., 1968. Cell to cell interaction in the immune response. II. The source of hemolysis-forming cells in irradiated mice given bone marrow and thymus or thoracic duct lymphocytes. J. Exp. Med. 128, 821–837.

Morgan, D.A., Ruscetti, F.W., Gallo, R., 1976. Selective in vitro growth of T lymphocytes from normal human bone marrows. Science 193, 1007–1008.

Moore, M.A.S., Owen, J.J.T., 1966. Experimental studies on the development of the bursa of Fabriciuus. Dev. Biol. 14, 401–451.

Mudd, S., 1932. A hypothetical mechanism of antibody formation. J. Immunol. 23, 423–427.

Nowell, P.C., 1960. Phytohemeagglutinin: an initiator of mitosis in cultures of normal human lymphocytes. Cancer Res. 20, 462–466.

Otto, R., 1906. Das Theobald Smithsche Phänomen der Serümüberempfindlichkeit. Von Leuthold Gedenkschrift 1, 153.

Padget, E.C., 1932. Is iso-grafting praticable ? Southern Med. J. 25, 895.

Pauling, L., 1940. A theory of the structure and process of formation of antibodies. J. Am. Chem. Soc. 62, 2643–2657.

Prehn, R.T., Main, J.M., 1957. Immunity to methylcholanthrene-induced sarcomas. J. Nat. Cancer Inst. 18, 769–778.

Raff, M.C., Sternberg, M., Taylor, R.B., 1970. Immunoglobulin determinants on the surface of mouse lymphoid cells. Nature 225, 553–554.

Roitt, I.M., Doniach, D., Campbell, P.N., Hudson, R.V., et al., 1956. Autoantibodies in Hashimoto's disease (lymphadenoid goiter). Lancet 2, 820–821.

Rose, N.R., Bona, C., 1993. Defining criteria for autoimmune diseases (witebsky's postulates revisited). Immunol. Today 14, 426–430.

Rose, N.R., Witebsky, E., 1956. Studies on organ specificity. V. Changes in the thyroid glands of rabbits following active immunization with rabbit thyroid extracts. J. Immunol. 76, 417–427.

Schwartz, R., Dameshek, W., 1960. The effects of 6-mercaptopurine on homografts reactions. J. Clin. Invest. 38, 952–958.

Schirrmacher, V., Rajewsky, K., 1970. Determination of antibody class in a system of cooperating antigenic determinants. J. Exp. Med. 132, 1019–1034.

Smith, T.H., 1905. Degrees of susceptibility to Diphteria toxin among guinea pigs. Transmission from parents to offspring. J. Med. Res. 13, 341–348.

Stutman, O., 1975. Chemical carcinogenesis in nude mice: comparison between nude mice from homogygous matings and heterozygous matings and effects of age and carcinogen dose. J. Nat. Cancer Inst. 62, 353–358.

Tauber, A.I., 1999. L'immunologia dell'io. Mc Graw Hill, Milano.

Thomas, L., 1959. Discussion. In: Lawrence, H.S. (Ed.), Cellular and Humoral Aspects of Hypersensitivity State. Hoeber, New York, p. 529.

Torrigiani, G., Doniach, D., Roitt, I.M., 1969. Serum thyroglobulin levels in healthy subjects and in patients with thyroid disease. J. Clin. Endocrinol. Metab. 29, 305–314.

Van Bekkum, D.W., Vos, O., 1957. Immunological aspects of homo-and heterologous bone marrow transplantation in irradiated animals. J. Cell. Physiol. 50 (suppl. 1), 139–156.

Van Der Bruggen, P., Traversari, C., Chomez, P., Lurquin, C., De Plaen, E., Van den Eynde, B., et al., 1991. A gene encoding an antigen recognized by cytolitic T lymphocytes on a human melanoma. Science 254, 1643–1647.

# FURTHER READING

Ada, G.L., Nossal, G., 1987. La teoria della selezione clonale. In: Celada, F. (Ed.), La nuova immunologia. Le Scienze Editore, Milano, pp. 30–37.

Balkwill, F., Mantovani, A., 2001. Inflammation and cancer. Back to Virchow ? Lancet 357, 539–545.

Billingham, R., Brent, L., Medawar, P.B., 1953. Actively acquired tolerance to foreign cells. Nature 172, 603–606.

Billingham, R., Brent, L., Medawar, P.B., 1956. Quantitative studies on tissue transplantation immunity. III. Actively acquired tolerance. Philos. Trans. Royal Soc. 239, 357–414.

Bonomo, L., Schena, F.P. (Eds.), 1979. Immunologia e immunoterapia. Dedalo, Bari.

Burgio, G.B., 1983. L'io biologico: questa nostra bioindividualità. Fed. Med. 36, 508–511.

Burnet, F.M., 1954. How antibodies are made. Sci. Am. 191, 74–78.

Burnet, F.M., 1968. Changing Patterns: An Atypical Biography. Heimemann, Sidney.

Burnet, F.M., 1970a. The concept of immunological surveillance. Prog. Exp. Tumor Res. 13, 1–27.

Burnet, F.M., 1970b. Immunological Surveillance. Pergamon Press, Oxford-London.

Cohn, M., 1972. Immunology: what are the rules of the game? Cell. Immunol. 5, 1–20.

Conley, M.E., 1994. X-linked immunodeficiences. Curr. Opin. Gen. Dev. 4, 401–406.

Coombs, R.R.A., Gell, P.G.H., 1963. The classification of allergic reactions responsible for allergic reactions underlying diseases. In: Gell, P.G.H., Coombs, R.R.A. (Eds.), Clinical Aspects of Immunology, 1963. Blackwell Scientific Publications, Oxford, p. 217.

Cooper, M.D., et al., 1966. The functions of the immune system and bursa system in the chicken. J. Exp. Med. 123, 76–93.

Corbellini, G., 1997. Le grammatiche del vivente. Storia della biologia molecolare. Laterza, Roma-Bari.

Croce, C.M., Nowell, P.C., 1986. Molecular genetics of human B cell neoplasia. Adv. Immunol. J. 38, 245–274.

Debré, P., 2000. Louis Pasteur. The John Hopkins University Press, Baltimore.

Dinarello, C.A., 1984. Interleukin-1. Rev. Inf. Diseases 6, 51–95.

Dunn, G.P., Bruce, A.T., Ikeda, H., Old, L.J., Schreiber, R.D., 2002. Cancer immunoediting: from immunosurveillance to tumor escape. Nat. Immunol. 3, 991–998.

Edelman, G.M., 1970. The structure and functions of antibodies. Sci. Am. 223, 34–42.

Edelman, G.M., 1971. Antibody structure and molecular immunology. Ann. N Y Acad. Sci. 190, 5–25.

Ehrlich, P., Morgenroth, J., 1899. Zur Theorie der Lysinwirkung. Berliner Klinische Wochenschrift 36, 481–486.

Fagraeus, A., 1948. Antibody production in relation to development of plasma cells. Acta Med. Scand. 130 (Suppl. 204), 3.

Fenner, F., 2006. Nature, Nurture and Chance: The Lives of Frank and Charles Fenner. Australian National University Press, Camberra.

Ferrata, A., 1907. Die Unwirksamkeit der Komplexen Hämolysine in salzfreinen Lösungen und ihre ursache. Die Berliner Klinische Wochenschrift 44, 366–368.

Fischer, A., 1993. Primary T-cell immunodeficiencies. Curr. Opin. Immunol. 5, 569–578.

Gibson, T., Medawar, P.B., 1943. The fate of skin homografts in man. J. Anat. 77, 229–310.

Gitlin, D., 1955. Low resistance to infection: relationship to abnormalities in gammaglobulin, 31, p. 359–365.

Glick, B., Chang, T.S., 1956. The bursa of Fabricius and antibody production. Poult. Sci. 35, 224.

Good, R.A., 1976. Runestones in immunology: inscriptions to journeys of discovery and analysis. J. Immunol. 117, 1413–1428.

Greaves, M.F., 1986. Differentiation-linked leukemogenesis in lymphocytes. Science 234, 697–704.

Haber, E., 1964. Recovery of antigenic specificity after denaturation and complete reduction of disulfides in papain fragments of antibody. Proc. Nat. Acad. Sci. USA 52, 1099–1106.

Hodgkin, P.D., Heath, W.R., Baxter, A.G., 2007. The clonal selection theory: 50 years since the revolution. Nat. Immunol. 8, 1019–1026.

Jenner, F., 1798. An Inquiry into Causes and Effects of Variolae Vaccinae, London.

Jerne, N.K., 1955. The natural selection theory of antibody formation. Proc. Nat. Acad. Sci. USA 41, 849–857.

Köhler, G., Milstein, C., 1975. Continuous cultures of fused cells secreting antibody of predefined species. Nature 256, 495–497.

Landsteiner, K., 1901. Ueber Agglutinationserscheinungen normalen menschlichen Blutes. Wiener Klinische Wochenschrift. 14, 1132–1134.

Landsteiner, K., 1921. Ueber heterogenetischen antigen und Hapten. Biochemische Zeitschrift 119, 294.

Landsteiner, K., 1945. The Specificity of Serological Reactions. Harvard University Press, Cambridge, MA.

Landsteiner, K., Chase, M.W., 1942. Experiments of transfer of cutaneous sensitivity to simple compounds. Proc. Soc. Exp. Biol. Med. 49, 668–690.

Lawrence, H.S., 1954. The transfer of generalized cutaneous hypersensitivity of delayed tuberculin type in man by means of the constituents of disrupeted leukocytes. J. Clin. Investigation 33, 951.

Mac Lean, L.D., Zak, S.J., Varco, R.L., Good, R.A., 1956. Thymic tumor and acquired agammaglobulinemia, a clinical and experimental study of the immune response. Surgery 40, 1010.

Mantovani, A., Sozzani, S., Locati, M., Allavena, P., 2002. Macrophage polarization: tumor-associated macrophages as a paradigm for polarized M2 mononuclear phagocytes. Trends Immunol. 23, 549–555.

Marrack, P., Kappler, J., Kotzin, B.L., 2001. Autoimmune disease: why and where it occurs. Nat. Med. 7, 899–905.

Metchnikoff, E., 1901. L'immunité dans les maladies infectieuses (résumé). Masson, Paris.

Moore, M.A.S., Owen, J.J.T., 1965. Chromosome marker studies on the development of the hemopoietic system in the chick embryo. Nature 208, 956.

Nossall, G.J., Ledeberg, J., 1958. Antibody production by single cells. Nature 181, 1419–1420.

Owen, J.J.T., Ritter, M.A., 1974. Tissue interaction in the development of thymus lymphocyte. J. Exp. Med. 129, 431–442.

Portier, P., Richet, C., 1902. De l'action anaphylactique de certains venins. Comptes Rendus des Sciences de la Société de Biologie 54, 170–172.

Roitt, I.M., 1969. The cellular basis of immunological responses. Lancet 2, 367.

Rosen, F.S., Cooper, M.D., Wedgwood, R.J., 1995. The primary immunodeficiences. New Engl. J. Med. 333, 431–440.

Sexton, C., 1999. Burnet: A Life. Oxford University Press, Melbourne.

Silverstein, A.M., 2009. A History of Immunology, second ed Academic Press, San Diego.

Soderqvist, T., 2003. Science Autobiography: The Troubled Life of Niels Jerne. Yale University Press, New Haven.

Talmage, D.W., 1957. Allergy and immunology. Ann. Rev. Med. 8, 239–256.

Tonegawa, S., 1983. Somatic generation of antibody diversity. Nature 302, 575–581.

Van Den Eynde, B.J., Van Der Bruggen, P., 1997. T cell defined tumor antigens. Curr. Opin. Immunol. 9, 684–693.

Von Pirquet, C., Schick, B., 1905. Die Serum Krankheit, Leipzig, Deutiche (Serum Sickness). Williams and Wilkins Co., Baltimore, 1951.

Witebski, E., Rose, N.R., 1956. Studies on organ specificity. IV. Production of rabbit thyroid antibodies in the rabbit. J. Immunol. 76, 408–416.

Witebsky, E., Rose, N.R., Terplan, K.K., Paine, J.R., Egan, R.W., 1957. Chronic thyroiditis and autoimmunization. J. Am. Med. Assoc. 164, 1439–1447.

Zinkernagel, R.M., Doherty, P.C., 1974a. Restriction of in vitro T cell-mediated cytotoxicity in lymphocytic choriomemngitis within a syngeneic or semiallagenic system. Nature 248, 701–702.

Zinkernagel, R.M., Doherty, P.C., 1974b. Immunological surveillance against altered self components by sensitized T lymphocytes in lymphocytic choriomeningitis. Nature 251, 547–548.

Printed in the United States
By Bookmasters